T0231183

# International Social Health Care Policy, Programs, and Studies

*International Social Health Care Policy, Programs, and Studies* has been co-published simultaneously as *Social Work in Health Care*, Volume 43, Numbers 2/3 2006.

# International Social Health Care Policy, Programs, and Studies

Gary Rosenberg, PhD
Andrew Weissman, PhD
Editors

*International Social Health Care Policy, Programs, and Studies* has been co-published simultaneously as *Social Work in Health Care*, Volume 43, Numbers 2/3 2006.

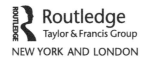

Routledge
Taylor & Francis Group
NEW YORK AND LONDON

First published by
The Haworth Press, Inc.
10 Alice Street
Binghamton, N Y 13904-1580

This edition published 2011 by Routledge

Routledge
Taylor & Francis Group
711 Third Avenue
New York, NY 10017

Routledge
Taylor & Francis Group
2 Park Square, Milton Park
Abingdon, Oxon OX14 4RN

*International Social Health Care Policy, Programs, and Studies* has been co-published simultaneously as *Social Work in Health Care,* Volume 43, Numbers 2/3 2006.

© 2006 by The Haworth Press, Inc. All rights reserved. No part of this work may be reproduced or utilized in any form or by any means, electronic or mechanical, including photocopying, microfilm and recording, or by any information storage and retrieval system, without permission in writing from the publisher.

The development, preparation, and publication of this work has been undertaken with great care. However, the publisher, employees, editors, and agents of The Haworth Press and all imprints of The Haworth Press, Inc., including The Haworth Medical Press® and The Pharmaceutical Products Press®, are not responsible for any errors contained herein or for consequences that may ensue from use of materials or information contained in this work. With regard to case studies, identities and circumstances of individuals discussed herein have changed to protect confidentiality. Any resemblence to actual persons, living or dead, is entirely coincidental.

The Haworth Press is committed to the dissemination of ideas and information according to the highest standards of intellectual freedom and the free exchange of ideas. Statements made and opinions expressed in this publication do not necessarily reflect the views of the Publisher, Directors, Management, or staff of The Haworth Press, Inc., or an endorsement by them.

Cover design by Lora Wiggins.

**Library of Congress Cataloging-in-Publication Data**

Doris Siegel Memorial Colloquim (9th : 2004 : Mount Sinai Medical Center) International Social Health Care Policy, Programs, and Studies/ Gary Rosenberg, Andrew Weissman, editors.
    p. cm.
    Papers presented at the Ninth Doris Siegel Memorial Colloquium held May 19-20, 2004 at the Mount Sinai Medical Center.
    "Co-published simultaneously as Social work in health care, volume 43, numbers 2/3 2006"
    Includes bibliographical references and index.
    ISBN 13: 978-0-7890-3347-5 (hard cover : alk. paper)
    ISBN 10: 0-7890-3347-X (hard cover : alk. paper)
    ISBN 13: 978-0-7890-3348-2 (soft cover : alk paper)
    ISBN 10: 0-7890-3348-8 (soft cover : alk. paper)
    1. Medical social work–Congresses. 2. Medical policy–Congresses. 3. Social medicine–Congresses. I. Rosenberg, Gary. II. Weissman, Andrew, 1941– III. Social work in health care. IV. Title.
HV687.D67 2004
362.1′0425–dc22
                                                         2006002960

# Monographs from *Social Work in Health Care*™

For additional information on these and other Haworth Press titles, including descriptions, tables of contents, reviews, and prices, use the QuickSearch catalog at http://www.HaworthPress.com.

1. *Advancing Social Work Practice in the Health Care Field: Emerging Issues and New Perspectives,* edited by Gary Rosenberg, PhD, and Helen Rehr, DSW (Vol. 8, No. 3, 1983). *"Excellent articles, useful bibliographies, and additional reading lists." (Australian Social Work)*

2. *Social Work and Genetics: A Guide to Practice,* edited by Sylvia Schild, DSW, and Rita Beck Black, DSW (Supplement #1, 1984). *"Precisely defines the responsibilities of social work in the expanding field of medical genetics and presents a clear, comprehensive overview of basic genetic principles and issues." (Health and Social Work)*

3. *Social Workers in Health Care Management: The Move to Leadership,* edited by Gary Rosenberg, PhD, and Sylvia S. Clarke, MSc, ACSW (Vol. 12, No. 3, 1988). *"Social workers interested in hospital social work management and the potential for advancement within the health care field will find the book interesting and challenging as well as helpful." (Social Thought)*

4. *The Changing Context of Social Health Care: Its Implications for Providers and Consumers,* edited by Helen Rehr, DSW, and Gary Rosenberg, PhD (Vol. 15, No. 4, 1991). *"Required reading for every student and practitioner with a vision of improving our health care delivery system." (Candyce S. Berger, PhD, MSW, Director of Social Work, University of Washington Medical Center; Associate Professor, School of Social Work, University of Washington)*

5. *Women's Health and Social Work: Feminist Perspectives,* edited by Miriam Meltzer Olson, DSW (Vol. 19, No. 3/4, 1994). *"[Chapters] explore how social workers can better understand and address women's health, including such conditions as breast cancer, menopause, and depression. They also discuss health care centers and African-American women and AIDS." (Reference & Research Book News)*

6. *Social Work in Ambulatory Care: New Implications for Health and Social Services,* edited by Gary Rosenberg, PhD, and Andrew Weissman, DSW (Vol. 20, No. 1, 1994). *"A most timely book dealing with issues related to the current shift in health care delivery to ambulatory care and social work's need to position itself in this health care arena." (Barbara Berkman, DSW, Director of Research and Quality Assessment, Massachusetts General Hospital; Associate Director, Harvard Upper New England Geriatric Education Center, Harvard Medical School)*

7. *Social Work Leadership in Healthcare: Directors' Perspectives,* edited by Gary Rosenberg, PhD, and Andrew Weissman, DSW (Vol. 20, No. 4, 1995). *Social work managers describe their work and work environment, detailing what qualities and traits are needed to be effective and successful now and in the future.*

8. *Social Work in Pediatrics,* edited by Ruth B. Smith, PhD, MSW, and Helen G. Clinton, MSW (Vol. 21, No. 1, 1995). *"It presents models of service delivery and clinical practice that offer responses to the challenges of today's health care system." (Journal of Social Work Education)*

9. *Professional Social Work Education and Health Care: Challenges for the Future,* edited by Mildred D. Mailick, DSW, and Phyllis Caroff, DSW (Vol. 24, No. 1/2, 1996). *Responds to critical concerns about the educational preparation of social workers within the rapidly changing health care environment.*

10. *Fundamentals of Perinatal Social Work: A Guide for Clinical Practice with Women, Infants, and Families,* edited by Regina Furlong Lind, MSW, LCSW, and Debra Honig Bachman, MSW, LCSW (Vol. 24, No. 3/4, 1997). *"A knowledge summation of the essence of perinatal social work that is long overdue. It is a must for any beginning perinatal social worker to own one!"*

*(Charlotte Collins Bursi, MSSW, Perinatal Social Worker, University of Tennessee Newborn Center; Founding President, National Association of Perinatal Social Workers)*

11. **International Perspectives on Social Work in Health Care: Past, Present and Future,** edited by Gail K. Auslander, DSW (Vol. 25, No. 1/2, 1997). *"The authors explore the need for new theoretical and practice models, in addition to developments in health and social work research and administration." (Council on Social Work and Education)*

12. **Social Work in Mental Health: Trends and Issues,** edited by Uri Aviram (Vol. 25, No. 3, 1997). *"Suggests ways to maintain social work values in a time that emphasizes cost containment and legal requirements that may result in practices and policies that are antithetical to the profession." (Phyllis Solomon, PhD, Professor, School of Social Work, University of Pennsylvania)*

13. **Behavioral Social Work in Health Care Settings,** edited by Gary Rosenberg, PhD, and Andrew Weissman, PhD (Vol. 31, No. 2, 2000). *"A Valuable Group of Research Studies examining important and pertinent issues. . . . Offers a fresh perspective on critical problems encountered by health care institutions, providers, patients, and families. Excellent." (Mildred D. Mailick, DSW, Professor Emerita, Hunter College School of Social Work, City University of New York)*

14. **Behavioral and Social Sciences in 21st Century Health Care: Contributions and Opportunities,** edited by Gary Rosenberg, PhD, and Andrew Weissman, PhD (Vol. 33, No. 1, 2001). *"Stimulating and Provocative. . . . The range of topics covered makes this book an ideal reader for health care practice courses with a combined health/mental health focus." (Goldie Kadushin, PhD, Associate Professor, School of Social Welfare, University of Wisconsin-Milaukee)*

15. **Clinical Data-Mining in Practice-Based Research: Social Work in Hospital Settings,** edited by Irwin Epstein, PhD, and Susan Blumenfield, DSW (Vol. 33, No. 3/4, 2001). *"Challenging and illuminating. . . . This remarkable collection of exemplary studies provides inspiration and support to social workers. This book will be valuable not only as a guide to practitioners, but also is an important addition to the teaching materials for courses in social work in health care and in social research methodology." (Kay V. Davidson, DSW, Dean and Professor, University of Connecticut School of Social Work, West Hartford)*

16. **Social Work Health and Mental Health: Practice, Research and Programs,** edited by Alun C. Jackson, PhD, and Steven P. Segal, PhD (Vol. 34, No. 1/2 and 3/4, 2001, and Vol. 35, No. 1/2, 2002). *Explores international perspectives on social work practice in health and mental health.*

17. **Social Work Visions from Around the Globe: Citizens, Methods, and Approaches,** edited by Anna Metteri, MSocSc, Teppo Kröger, PhD, Anneli Pohjola, PhD, and Pirkko-Liisa Rauhala, Dr. Habil, DSW (Vol. 39, No. 1/2 and 3/4, 2004). *"VALUABLE to practitioners in health and mental health. . . . Shows in a practical way how citizenship can be an inclusive practice related to social justice, rather than a way of excluding people from opportunities and resources in our societies." (Heather D' Cruz, PhD, MSW, Senior Lecturer in Social Work,, School of Health and Social Development, Faculty of Health and Behavioral Sciences, Deakin University, Geelong, Victoria, Australia)*

18. **Bibliometrics in Social Work,** edited by Gary Holden, DSW, Gary Rosenberg, PhD, and Kathleen Barker, PhD (Vol. 41, No. 3/4, 2005). *An overview of the pros and cons of using bibliometrics in social work research.*

19. **The Geometry of Care: Linking Resources, Research, and Community to Reduce Degrees of Separation Between HIV Treatment and Prevention,** edited by Debbie Indyk, PhD (Vol. 42, No. 3/4, 2006). *An examination of ways to link bottom-up and top-down activities to further care, services, resources, training, theory, and policy analysis for AIDS treatment and prevention.*

20. **International Social Health Care Policy, Programs, and Studies,** edited by Gary Rosenberg, PhD, and Andrew Weissman, PhD (Vol. 43, No. 2/3, 2006). *"Exemplifies how social work attempts to understand and respond creatively to the specific social issues of different countries from a clinical, programmatic and policy perspectives. . . . Contributors are experts in their respective areas of work and share their views and experiences through this wonderful book." (Dr. Daniel Fu Keung Wong, PhD, Associae Professor, Department of Social Work and Social Administration, The University of Hong Kong)*

# International Social Health Care Policy, Programs, and Studies

## CONTENTS

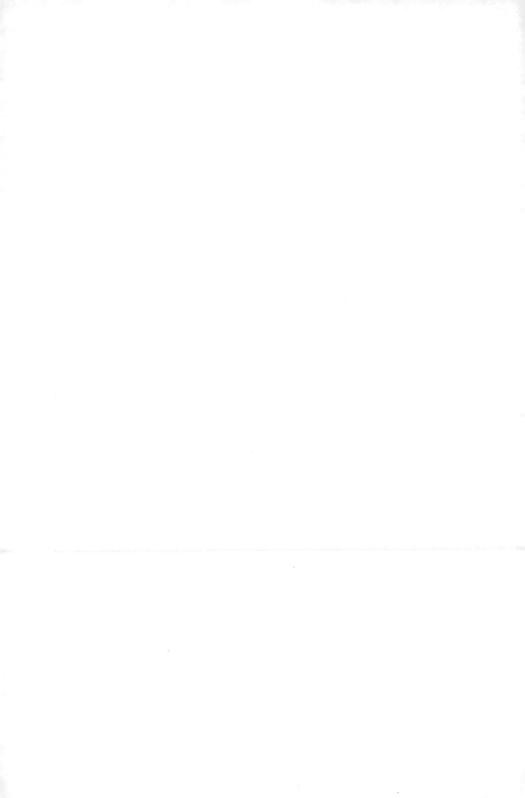

# ABOUT THE EDITORS

**Gary Rosenberg, PhD,** is currently the Edith J. Baerwald Professor of Community Medicine and Preventive Medicine, and Chairman of the Division of Social Work and Behavioral Science at the Mount Sinai School of Medicine. His previous position was as Executive Vice President of the Mount Sinai Medical Center and he was a member of the senior management staff for 28 years.

Dr. Rosenberg is the recipient of numerous awards, among them are the Outstanding Alumni Award from Hunter College and Adelphi University, and the Founders Day Award from New York University. He is a fellow of the New York Academy of Medicine and a member of the Social Work Pioneers Group.

Dr. Rosenberg maintains an active role on non-profit boards and is the President of the Board of the Center for Social Administration, a post-master's management education institute, President of the Board of Senior Health Partners, an agency serving the aging population of New York and a member of the Board of Directors of Union Settlement and Job Path, an agency serving mentally retarded and developmentally disabled adults.

Dr. Rosenberg is the Editor-in-Chief of two peer-reviewed journals on health policy and practices and on mental health. He has written or edited 12 books, 22 book chapters and is the author of over 60 articles in professional peer reviewed journals.

**Andrew Weissman, PhD,** is Associate Professor at The Mount Sinai School of Medicine in the Department of Community and Preventive Medicine, Division of Social Work and Behavioral Science. He received his AB from Antioch College, his MA in social work from the University of Chicago, and his PhD in social work from the University of Maryland.

Previously Dr. Weissman was the Director of the Department of Social Work Services of the Mount Sinai Hospital, Executive Vice President of Altro Health and Rehabilitation Services, and Director of the

United States Steel Counseling Center in Chicago, one of this country's first Employee Assistance Programs. He is the Managing Editor of the *Social Work in Health Care* journal and the co-editor of the *Social Work in Mental Health* journal.

Dr. Weissman has also received the prestigious Ida M. Cannon award of the Society for Social Work Directors in Health Care of The American Hospital Association. He is the author of numerous articles on social work in professional journals.

# Welcome to the Ninth Doris Siegel Memorial Fund Colloqium

Gary Rosenberg, PhD

As the Executive Secretary of the Doris Siegel Memorial Fund it is my pleasure to welcome you to the Ninth Doris Siegel Memorial Fund Colloquium. The focus of this Colloquium in the past has been on the interface between medicine, social work and other health professions. This year the planning Committee decided to focus on social work and global health issues. As the economies of all countries have become inter-dependent, travel has become a way of life. There is increasingly an interface among the countries of the world. The United Nations and voluntary organizations and for profit organizations are all focusing their efforts towards understanding towards global health issues and problems faced by us all. None of us can escape or close off our borders to health problems experienced by others around the world. There are numerous global health goals; clearly we all subscribe to reducing the excessive morality and morbidity suffered by the poor. We are all involved in countering potential threats resulting from economic crisis on healthy environments and risky behaviors. Each of our countries wishes to develop more effective health systems and we must expand the knowledge base and provide those tools for continuing gains into the 21st century. Social work has a huge role to play in helping to ameliorate the leading global risk factors. Let me briefly state there are

[Haworth co-indexing entry note]: "Welcome to the Ninth Doris Siegel Memorial Fund Colloqium." Rosenberg, Gary. Co-published simultaneously in *Social Work in Health Care* (The Haworth Press, Inc.) Vol. 43, No. 2/3, 2006, pp. 1-3; and: *International Social Health Care Policy, Programs, and Studies* (ed: Gary Rosenberg, and Andrew Weissman) The Haworth Press, Inc., 2006, pp. 1-3. Single or multiple copies of this article are available for a fee from The Haworth Document Delivery Service [1-800-HAWORTH, 9:00 a.m. - 5:00 p.m. (EST). E-mail address: docdelivery@haworthpress.com].

Available online at http://swhc.haworthpress.com
© 2006 by The Haworth Press, Inc. All rights reserved.
doi:10.1300/J010v43n02_01

three million childhood deaths each year because children are under weight. The fourth biggest cause of death in the world is unsafe sex, mostly HIV and AIDS but 40 million people infected, 28 million of them in Africa. Hypertension, overweight and obesity, consumption of fatty, sugary and salty foods raises risks. At least 220,000 people in the United States and Canada and 320,000 people in Western Europe die each year from these factors. Iron deficiency affects 2 billion people and causes a million deaths each year. Indoor air pollution, the burning of solid waste from cooking and heating, causes 36% of all respiratory infections and 22% of all chronic pulmonary diseases in the world. Unsafe waters, sanitation and hygiene account for 1.7 million deaths and alcohol consumption 1.8 million. Psychological, social and environmental issues inherent in these leading risk factors are the day to day life of social workers around the world. Social workers advocate for broad based interventions that would make available reproductive decisions and free access to reproductive health information and contraception basic education especially for women, aid to escape proverty, environmental programs all designed to improve conditions in poor countries while reducing consumption in those countries that are mine fortunate. We must also improve global systems for disease surveillance these must be comprehensive and transparent, capable of measuring the burdens of disease, detect new and emerging problems, track changes in disease incidents and prevalence. The World Health Organization has targeted protection of the child environment, preventive interventions to reduce incidents of HIV infection, attempt to reduce risks associated with cardiovascular disease, primarily salt and cholesterol lowing strategies and to increase the role of government in influences behaviors such as government taxes on tobacco and control of salt content in processed foods. Social work and public health advocates have supported risk prevention policies that focus on populations rather then aiming at high-risk individuals. The programs which are primary rather then secondary prevention and programs that control distal rather than proximal risks to health. That is, focusing on education and poverty can yield fundamental and sustain improvements to future health status. Social work is an important partner is such efforts. We are gathered together and will be hearing from social workers around the world who are providing creative programmatic responses to needs of populations of people and segments of populations in their respective countries. Many of the social workers you will hear from today and tomorrow have had an association and an affiliation with The Mount Sinai Medical Center. We have benefited from that collaboration, as have they. In many ways it is an example of the kind of cooperation and exchange that must go on in order to achieve the goals of improving the global health status. It is the hope of the Planning Committee that our conference today will make a small contribution to the knowledge base of social work by exchanging our best practices, our most creative programs and our technologies for teaching, servicing our client population and evaluating the effects of what we do.

# The Ninth Doris Siegel Memorial Conference Tribute

Helen Rehr, DSW

Welcome. This is the Ninth Doris Siegel Memorial Colloquium, since her death over 30 years ago. Most of you will not have known her. We memorialize her because of what she has left us, her accomplishments, her values and her advocacy on behalf of social-health issues–within this institution, in the broader communities and on the national scene.

Doris came to Sinai in 1953 and remained until her death 18 years later. She was the Director of Social Work Services, and also the Edith J. Baerwald Professor of Community Medicine, the only endowed chair in social work in a medical institution. She also served as the Chairperson of the Division of Social Work.

Doris was a pragmatist. She related to theory and scientific knowledge, but would always start with questions "what does it mean?" and "will it enhance practice and program?" In 1956 Doris Siegel and Dr. Martin Steinberg, Mount Sinai's beloved illustrious CEO, published a joint article in *Hospitals* asking, "is social work a luxury or necessity?" The article stated "it reasonable to assume that hospitals would subscribe to our conclusion that social services must be placed high on the priority list if a hospital is to render service which is not only useful but complete." Their projections extended social work in medical institu-

Helen Rehr, DSW, is Professor Emerita of Community Medicine (Social Work), The Mount Sinai School of Medicine, City University of New York.

[Haworth co-indexing entry note]: "The Ninth Doris Siegel Memorial Conference Tribute." Rehr, Helen. Co-published simultaneously in *Social Work in Health Care* (The Haworth Press, Inc.) Vol. 43, No. 2/3, 2006, pp. 5-7; and: *International Social Health Care Policy, Programs, and Studies* (ed: Gary Rosenberg, and Andrew Weissman) The Haworth Press, Inc., 2006, pp. 5-7. Single or multiple copies of this article are available for a fee from The Haworth Document Delivery Service [1-800-HAWORTH, 9:00 a.m. - 5:00 p.m. (EST). E-mail address: docdelivery@haworthpress.com].

Available online at http://swhc.haworthpress.com
© 2006 by The Haworth Press, Inc. All rights reserved.
doi:10.1300/J010v43n02_02

tions and set the philosophy that care was not just physical care, but social health as well. She created a unique place for social work in social-health services, in education and in research–always working collaboratively with health care colleagues. She saw illness and disorders in larger context of one's family, environment and its effect on quality of life. She brought humanism and science together. She was a brilliant administrator, selecting the best professionals and always crediting them for their ideas and performance. She was creative. One worked *with* her (not *for* her), learning and becoming strengthened by her convictions: her fearlessness in tackling meaningful issues, and her continual furthering of innovative ideas. She was community-sensitive, knowing that an institution must go beyond its walls. When she was inducted into the Baerwald Chair in 1969 she said social work and medicine have a responsibility for "reaching out more aggressively not only to those we serve, but to those whom we should serve."

She had a personal warmth, compassion and grace, with a critical interest in people. She loved having people around her. She was a gracious hostess. I remembered my mother who after being invited to dinner–in contrasting to her own daughter's dinners said "that Doris she sets a fine table."

Her commitment to Mount Sinai was boundary-less. She saw its potential for the best social-health care. Today, we at Mount Sinai have become a large health system. We see its progressive directions in many areas such as a nationally recognized geriatric social-health center, a comprehensive pediatric center, a range of specialty surgical and medical concentrations, and much more–all reflecting a high quality of medical services with commitment to the psychosocial needs of their patients–plus a medical school developing an innovative curriculum in which students are being groomed to deal with a fast changing health care, yet, still valuing the doctor-patient relationship. Doris would be proud of the innovative programs.

Innovative programs benefiting our patients are essential in a changing health care environment. I don't have to tell this audience that in a climate of managed care, sharp reductions in reimbursement, and downsizing, medical institutions, which project themselves as 'corporate entities,' introduce a more for less philosophy and talk of 'products' rather than care, have shifted from being a voluntary social utility to a commercialized industry.

In an insurance managed care environment, health professionals lose the option to set standards. To be a quality and even a cost-effective institution requires a trust among those who provide and receive services. Dr. Jeremiah Barondess, Director of the New York Academy of Medicine says "the social responsibility of medicine is an old mandate (needing to be) renewed today as health care faces a critical watershed." Doris would have said "what we need is to return to social justice and equity."

This is the Ninth Colloquium. In each of the past eight, the subjects have been current, meaningful and frequently a "first" in public deliberations. These Colloquia have dealt with: inter-professionalism, values and ethical dilemmas, milestones in social work and medicine and their meaning for the future, problems and solutions to access, and the changing context of social work in ambulatory care. Today the subject is "International Social Health Care: Policy, Program and Studies."

I know it would be meaningful and will continue to honor the qualities Doris so fully embodied.

# The Strength-Focused
# and Meaning-Oriented Approach
# to Resilience and Transformation (SMART):
# A Body-Mind-Spirit Approach
# to Trauma Management

Cecilia L. W. Chan, PhD
Timothy H. Y. Chan, BCogSc
Siv Man Ng, RCMP

**SUMMARY.** This article introduces the Strength-focused and Mean-ing-oriented Approach to Resilience and Transformation (SMART) as a model of crisis intervention, which aims at discovering inner strengths

Cecilia L. W. Chan is Professor, Department of Social Work and Social Adminis-tration and Director, Centre on Behavioral Health, the University of Hong Kong. Tim-othy H. Y. Chan is Research Coordinator, and Siv Man Ng is Clinical Coordinator, Centre on Behavioral Health, the University of Hong Kong.

Address correspondence to: Cecilia L. W. Chan, PhD, Director, Centre on Behav-ioral Health, G/F, Pauline Chan Building, 10 Sassoon Road, Pokfulam, Hong Kong (E-mail: cecichan@hku.hk).

The authors would also like to acknowledge the participation of the subjects in this study and to thank Mr. Hang-Sau Ng and Miss Jenny Lau of the Community Rehabili-tation Network of the Hong Kong Society for Rehabilitation for their active participa-tion in the evaluation study of the SMART intervention for people with chronic illness in the aftermath of community trauma of SARS.

Part of this paper was presented at the 9th Doris Siegel Colloquium at Mount Sinai Medical University, New York on the 19th of May, 2004.

[Haworth co-indexing entry note]: "The Strength-Focused and Meaning-Oriented Approach to Resil-ience and Transformation (SMART): A Body-Mind-Spirit Approach to Trauma Management." Chan, Cecilia L. W., Timothy H. Y. Chan, and Siv Man Ng. Co-published simultaneously in *Social Work in Health Care* (The Haworth Press, Inc.) Vol. 43, No. 2/3, 2006, pp. 9-36; and: *International Social Health Care Policy, Programs, and Studies* (ed: Gary Rosenberg, and Andrew Weissman) The Haworth Press, Inc., 2006, pp. 9-36. Single or multiple copies of this article are available for a fee from The Haworth Document Delivery Service [1-800-HAWORTH, 9:00 a.m. - 5:00 p.m. (EST). E-mail address: docdelivery@haworthpress.com].

Available online at http://swhc.haworthpress.com
© 2006 by The Haworth Press, Inc. All rights reserved.
doi:10.1300/J010v43n02_03

through meaning reconstruction. Limitations of conventional crisis management and current findings in post-traumatic growth research are discussed. Instead of adopting a pathological framework, the SMART approach holds a holistic view of health, employs facilitative strategies, and promotes dynamic coping. Intervention components include Eastern spiritual teachings, physical techniques such as yoga and meditation, and psycho-education that promotes meaning reconstruction. Efficacy of the SMART model is assessed with reference to two pilot studies conducted in Hong Kong at the time when the SARS pandemic caused widespread fear and anxiety in the community. Response to potential criticisms of the SMART model is attempted. *[Article copies available for a fee from The Haworth Document Delivery Service: 1-800-HAWORTH. E-mail address: <docdelivery@haworthpress.com> Website: <http://www.HaworthPress.com> © 2006 by The Haworth Press, Inc. All rights reserved.]*

**KEYWORDS.** Trauma, resilience, transformation, SARS, meaning reconstruction, strength-focused intervention, CISD, body-mind-spirit

## *LIFE AS A SERIES OF CRISES AND TRAUMATIC EXPERIENCES*

Life can be compared to a hurdle race with an uneven distribution of obstacles. As medical advances continue to stretch the human lifespan, it is increasingly more likely that we will meet more of these hurdles. Along the ever-lengthening running track, some of the typical obstacles that we might have to leap over are described below.

*Personal threats.* Over the last century, our victories over many infectious diseases were marked by a sharp decline in death rates (Ray, 2004). Ironically, as people live longer today, incidence of cancer and other degenerative diseases is currently on the rise. Moreover, thanks to earlier diagnosis and more effective treatments, individuals with incurable diseases such as HIV/AIDS can drastically extend their life expectancies. In effect, a growing population is now living with chronic medical conditions. Survivors have to cope with the aftermath of the diseases and of the sometimes invasive treatments.

*Relational threats.* The loss of a loved one, although inevitable for most individuals during their lifetime, can trigger distress and other health consequences (Parkes, 1996). Bereaved spouses have a higher incidence of heart disease and an increased risk of mortality within the first year of bereavement (Friedman, 2002; Ray, 2004). In a subtler sense of loss, the dissolution of relationships due to breakup, divorce or job loss can be equally traumatic. Individuals may become trapped in a state of bitterness and rage (Hung, Kung, & Chan, 2003). People grieving for personal losses are posed with the challenge to reconstruct their altered subjective world (Neimeyer, 2000).

*Social threats.* Events such as outbreaks of disease, terrorist attacks, or natural disasters not only are destructive in a physical sense, but also can cause invisible damage to public mental health. The anxiety and anger that result from natural forces or human acts do not dissipate quickly. Contributing to this widespread traumatization is the advent of technology that both shortens the delay and broadens the scope of information dissemination, which includes news on disasters and atrocities. As a number of studies on the impact of the September 11 terrorist attacks reveal, prolonged exposure to violent incidents in the media can lead to vicarious traumatization (Schlenger et al., 2002; Schuster et al., 2001). Frequent vicarious observations of atrocities and misfortune can induce a strong sense of vulnerability.

## CONVENTIONAL TRAUMA MANAGEMENT

Under the perceived threats of possible traumas, people naturally respond by becoming defensive. On the alert for any signs of harm, people are prone to activate their rigid mechanism of fight or flight. Translated into a social context, that means aggression or isolation. Although such responses are life preserving under imminent threats, indiscriminate applications of the friend-or-foe mentality are likely to generate maladaptive reactions, such as prolonged fear, anxiety and rigidity, which can fuel further conflicts. This negative energy resulted can be expressed either by depression or by aggression. Figure 1 shows the quadrants of the extreme reactions that people might display during crisis situations. Indulging in their suffering, people may isolate themselves or adopt measures such as suicide and self-harm; blaming the world, on the other hand, can lead to religious or political fanaticism.

Social work interventions take on the mission to assist people during their difficult times. In doing so, however, the social work profession–and related disciplines of medicine, psychology, and public administration as well–operates mainly within a pathology-based framework, which is geared toward the removal of symptoms and the revival of functioning to a pre-crisis level. Facing a client in distress, a

FIGURE 1. Extreme actions during a crisis

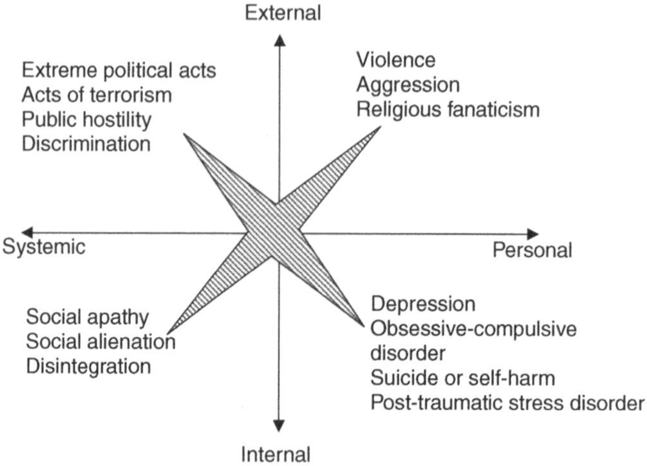

social worker is often like a handyman with a bag of tools who is looking for broken parts to fix. With a hammer at hand, everything around looks like a nail: a population is underprivileged, a family is dysfunctional, and an individual is vulnerable. The success of social work intervention is then measured by the number of problems that are identified in the client during intake and subsequently solved by the social worker by the time the client is discharged. As a result, short-term, solution-focused intervention models have largely replaced previously long-term, open-ended engagements. Direct practice has become an endeavor of reaching down and salvaging vulnerable people from all sorts of personal predicaments and social injustices. The key objectives are to identify vulnerabilities and to apply remedial patchwork.

## *CRISIS DEBRIEFING AND ITS APPLICATION*

Similar to psychology, which as a discipline saw marked development after World War II, the study of crisis debriefing originated from the concern of stress reactions that were exhibited by Vietnam war veterans. Although the scholarly quest of posttraumatic stress disorders (PTSD) is not one without confusion or controversy (Lamprecht & Sack, 2002), there has been remarkable progress on the appreciation of human reactions under trauma, the understanding of the causes of PTSD, and the development of prevention and treatment regimes (O'Shea, 2001). With the aim of neutralizing any negative repercussions that may follow a traumatic experience, conventional interventions for traumatized individuals see personal growth after trauma as complimentary at best, irrelevant at worst. For decades numerous psychosocial intervention models have been developed, among which one popular form is the Critical Incident Stress Debriefing (CISD, Mitchell & Everly, 2000). It has been applied to such a broad extent that its use is reported in a wide range of professions and populations, such as healthcare workers (Lane, 1993), firefighters (Mitchell, Schiller, Eyler, & Everly, 1999), murder investigators (Sewell, 1993), mortuary workers (Peterson, Nicolas, McGraw, Englert, & Blackman, 2002), police officers (Carlier, Voerman, & Gersons, 2000), and prisoners (Stoll & Edwards, 2002). Attempts were also made to provide a blanket psychological intervention for every exposed individual within a month of the September 11, 2001 attack (Miller, 2002).

Despite its popularity, recent research on the efficacy of the CISD has produced mixed results (Carlier, 2000; Everly & Boyle, 1999; Rose, Brewin, Andrews, & Kirk, 1999; van Emmerik, Kamphuis, Hulsbosch, & Emmelkamp, 2002). In some of the studies, people who received the debriefing were found to exhibit more PTSD symptoms subsequently than those who did not (e.g., Carlier et al., 2000), which raises concerns about re-traumatization during the debriefing process. Critics of the model argue that applying the debriefing indiscriminately to every individual after crisis may pathologize normal reactions under distress. Unnecessary remedial intervention, as Bonanno (2004) points out, may undermine or interfere with the natural course of human coping. More research is needed to better understand why some benefit from professional intervention and some do not. Moreover, in light of the growing body of literature on post-traumatic growth, it is time for social workers to devise methods to help clients not only to recover from the aftermath of crisis and trauma, but also to thrive in the process.

## *FROM TRAUMA TO GROWTH*

Not everyone reacts to adversities in the same way. Some people are more resilient than others. Whereas one individual may succumb to a morbid state, the other may flourish and grow from painful events (Schneider, 1994). Like other cultures in the world, the Chinese have developed their own understanding of hardship and suffering. The Chinese word for "trauma" (*chuangshang*) is the juxtaposition of two characters: "creation" (*chuang*) and "hurt" (*shang*). Traumatic experiences can create opportunities for growth by introducing fresh perspectives to one's life. Through this process, a person's emotional and spiritual capacities can be enhanced. Of course the Chinese culture does not deny the presence of pain and distress in people's experiences; rather, it is believed that distress and growth are not mutually exclusive. There is an old Chinese adage that says, "bitterness is the best medicine."

In this vein, people who experience traumatic events can be helped by casting their painful experiences in a more positive light. Once such a shift in focus is achieved, the course of the coping process can be shortened. From our clinical experience, the realization that traumatic experiences may lead to positive gains can be consoling to people in pain.

Although the fact that positive change can come from traumatic experiences has long been recognized in art and literature, it is not until recently that human service professionals saw the need for the scientific study of such a phenomenon. The term *transformation* was first systematically used to refer to positive post-trauma consequences by Tedeschi and Calhoun (1995), who documented numerous accounts of growth after traumatic events. Over the last decade, psychologists begin to recognize trauma as an opportunity for an individual to transform his or her own life. If people can maximize their learning from living through a traumatic experience, they may be rewarded by an increased awareness or even enlightenment (Schaefer & Moos, 1998, 2001). Qualitative accounts have been collated in the literature to provide a clearer typology of post-traumatic growth in various types of crisis. For example, one meta-analysis summarizes the current research in cancer survivors into three areas in which positive changes can occur (Thornton, 2002):

1. *Life perspective.* People reported a greater appreciation of life, a revision of life priorities, and an increased awareness of the importance of emotional and physical well-being.
2. *Interpersonal relationships.* People realized that relationships with others were more important, and reported an improvement in such relationships.
3. *Self.* People reported feeling a greater inner strength and independence, and discovered a greater self-respect and an improved self-image.

Changes in the area of self-conception in particular have attracted debate, because the findings are so far unclear. As Thornton (2002) points out, traumatized individuals may report self-derogation and increased vulnerability, but at the same time they might also describe a sense of mastery and self-esteem during the process of recovery and adaptation. We observe similar self-reports of victimization among our clients, but when they are asked about how they cope, they are able to share stories of their resilience and survivorship.

To investigate the possible pathways that lead to post-traumatic growth, Linley and Joseph (2004) review 39 empirical studies that document positive changes following trauma and adversity. The review indicates that coping styles, positive effects and optimism are all associated with growth. In the long run, people who report and maintain growth are less distressed subsequently (Linley & Joseph, 2004).

## *PROMOTING GROWTH IN CRISIS AS A SOCIAL WORKER*

Despite the promising findings in psychology literature, advocating growth-promoting practices in the hectic world of social work can be confusing at first glance. Part of the reason is that the scope of social work intervention can range widely from the remedial to the transcendental. Many social workers work under immense pressure as they spend most of their time struggling with the problems of their clients at the basic level. Although attending to the psychosocial needs and holistic well-being of clients seems to be vital, some social workers may find it to be a luxury under high caseload pressure.

Nevertheless, the past decade has seen the rise of a strength-focused perspective in the social work profession which objects to the obsession with victimhood and psychopathology, and which aims at more than getting everything "back to normal" (Graybeal, 2001; Saleebey, 1996). The *strengths perspective*, of which Dennis Saleebey (1999) is one of the forerunners, shifts the focus from pathology to strength and resilience. A social worker should look for strengths in people and resources in the environment. Of course, the symptoms and problems are very real, and so are the pain and suffering, but, as Saleebey (1999) argues, "it is as wrong to deny the possible as it is to deny the problem" (p. 15). The strengths perspective advocates an evolution in social work practice that puts clients in a more active role toward self-actualization. By working as a collaborator, the social worker not only heals the wound but facilitates growth and resilience, however dire or debilitating the client's situation may at first glance seem.

The strengths perspective has been applied to different fields of social work practice–gerontological social work (Chapin & Cox, 2001; Sullivan & Fisher, 1994), mental health (Rapp, 1998; Russo, 1999), community (Pollio, McDonald, & North, 1996), substance abuse (Moxley & Washington, 2001; Walker & Lee, 1998), and medical settings (Chazin, Kaplan, & Terio, 2000; Rowlands, 2001). In the area of crisis management, although there have been calls for a more strength-focused reformulation of crisis intervention to help positive changes after trauma (Fraser, 1998), a concrete framework is yet to be established. We envision a model of crisis intervention that will bring harmony for people undergoing crises (Figure 2). When devising a strength-focused crisis intervention, however, some specific questions have to be answered:

- how do we incorporate strength-focused intervention techniques in a time-limited group debriefing setting?
- how do we indigenize our intervention model in working with culturally diverse clients?
- how do we address physical and spiritual well-being, in the face of mounting evidence that confirms the link between physical and mental health?
- how do we know if it works or not?

FIGURE 2. Harmony after crisis resolution

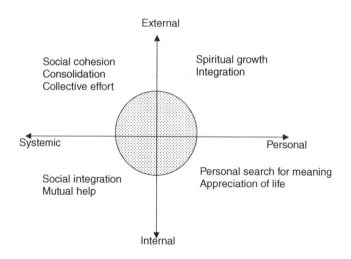

# STRENGTH-FOCUSED AND MEANING-ORIENTED APPROACH TO RESILIENCE AND TRANSFORMATION

In this article, we introduce a crisis intervention approach called the Strength-focused and Meaning-oriented Approach to Resilience and Transformation (SMART). Through time-limited contacts (ranging from one whole-day training to six weekly meetings) in a group setting, the SMART intervention attempts to foster growth in people undergoing crisis. The intervention process focuses at the rediscovery of self and the development of inner strength. The purpose of the SMART intervention, as stated in its name, is the attainment of resilience and transformation. The dual goals are two sides of the same coin: resilience pertains to resistance against the disruptions of normal functioning in the face of a crisis (Bonanno, 2004), and transformation describes the ability to grow in the aftermath of it (Tedeschi & Calhoun, 1995).

The emphasis on the meaning-making process partly reflects the latest development in grief research. According to Neimeyer (2001), finding and redefining the meanings of life during a major trauma is not merely a coping strategy, but is also a pathway to positive transformation. As Zebrack (2000) concludes in a qualitative study on the quality of life of leukemia and lymphoma survivors, "[the] quality of life outcomes partially may be a function of the cognitive frame or meaning that survivors attribute to their experience" (p. 39). In order to make sense of the traumatic experience, people often have to adjust their existing worldview. The assumptive world model that is posed by Janoff-Bulman (1989) is useful in explaining the significance of worldview to people experiencing trauma: an individual who is violated by traumatic events has to rebuild their assumptions of the world (e.g., whether it is a just world or not), especially those related to the purpose of life. Reframing a coherent worldview can be seen as a successful coping of the trauma. There appears to be empirical support for this in the study of cancer survivors, which shows that the quality of life of cancer survivors partly hinges on the outcome of the meaning-making process. Survivors who are still struggling to find a meaning in life have a poorer quality of life (Tomich & Helgeson, 2002), and those who have a sense of purpose display less psychological distress and better emotional and social functioning (Vickberg et al., 2001).

## THE SARS PANIC:
## AN APPLICATION OF THE SMART INTERVENTION

To explore how the SMART intervention can be applied in a crisis situation, a couple of intervention studies were conducted by the authors between April and September 2003 when Hong Kong was still struggling with the aftermath of an epidemic. The outbreak of Severe Acute Respiratory Syndrome (SARS) in March 2003 caught the world off guard. The disease, caused by a hitherto unknown strain of the corona virus, affected a number of countries across different continents. Apart from its fatality, currently estimated at about 15%, this new disease was especially threatening in several ways (World Health Organization, 2003). It has no vaccine and no treatment, the initial symptoms are non-specific and common, and the incubation period is long enough to allow both local and international transmission. Being the epicenter of the disease, Hong Kong had the second highest number of confirmed cases in the world (1,755 as of May 31, 2003, resulting in 299 deaths, HKSAR Department of Health, 2003). The outbreak had caused high levels of diffused general anxiety across society. In a community-wide survey that was conducted in May 2003, many respondents reported that they were worried about SARS, had developed sleeping problems, and could not concentrate properly (Hong Kong Mood Disorders Center, 2003a). Seldom was there a large scale crisis that can cause widespread distress and fear in the community. The SMART intervention, as explicated in the subsequent sections, can prove to be effective in helping people to deal with their posttraumatic stress.

## PRINCIPLES OF SMART INTERVENTION

The SMART intervention is an adaptation of the Eastern Body-Mind-Spirit (BMS) model that is developed by our research team. The BMS model relies heavily on Eastern philosophies and concepts drawn from Traditional Chinese Medicine to address the physical, mental, and spiritual needs of an individual. Since the 1990s, the BMS model has been widely used in Hong Kong in working with patients who are suffering from cancer, stroke, systemic lupus erythematosis, rheumatoid arthritis, diabetes, with people who are bereaved, infertile couples and divorced single mothers (Chan, Chan, Law, Wong, & Yu, 1998; Chan, Chow et al., 1996; Chan, Ho, Ng, & Chau, 1996; Lee, 1995; Man, 1996). Pilot trials have also been run in other Asian cities such as Singa-

pore and Beijing, where divorced women learn how to cope with
marital breakdowns (Chan, Fan, & Gong, 2003).

Based on the BMS framework, the SMART intervention is tailored
for people who are undergoing acute crises. The main characteristics of
the SMART intervention include the following:

*Integrative, multi-modal approaches.* The machinery of mainstream
psychotherapy is built upon skilled verbal exchanges between client
and counselor. Although this is an invaluable part of the therapy, a
wider variety of communication models should be explored. This is particularly necessary for clients who are cognitively less sophisticated and
verbally less articulate in the sharing of their emotions (Chan & Rhind,
1997). In addition, people coming from a culture which merits controlled emotional expression (e.g., Chinese, see Russell & Yik, 1996;
Tsai & Levenson, 1997) often refrain from talking openly about their
deepest emotions. Nonetheless, verbal communication is not the only
way people cope with their stress; psychologists are becoming increasingly aware of the idiosyncratic and creative ways of coping. Take
'grief work' as an example; the overt expression of sad emotions has
been traditionally seen as the key to adaptive coping in the West. The
absence of such expression in a grief situation may be regarded as a
form of repressed, delayed grief of which the person is in denial. In recent years, however, researchers have looked at bereaved people who
do not outwardly express grief and have found no pathological consequences in the long run (Bonanno, Keltner, Holen, & Horowitz, 1995;
Stroebe, Stroebe, Schut, Zech, & van den Bout, 2002). Despite the multifaceted nature of the human coping process (Bonanno, 2004), conventional posttraumatic intervention is limited by its over-reliance on the
verbal communication of grief. The danger of relying on a narrow set of
therapeutic strategies or arrogantly prescribing a single mode of coping
to every client cannot be overstated. Non-verbal channels of exchange,
therefore, should also be sought, experimented with, and consistently
incorporated into regular social work intervention. In crisis management, there have been attempts to introduce art in CISD intervention
(Morgan & White, 2003). The use of physical movement (Robbins,
1998) and meditation (Wolfsdorf & Zlotnick, 2001) for people experiencing trauma are also examples of this kind of multi-modal intervention.

The SMART intervention, which is guided by the principle that the
mind and body constitutes the synthetic whole of a person, incorporates
physical components (movement, breathing, massage, etc.) that can

bring about emotional changes. By borrowing ideas from Chinese forms of exercise (*tai-chi* movements) and Traditional Chinese Medicine (acupressure), the SMART intervention explores the possibility of formulating interventions that best reflect the Chinese holistic view of well-being.

*Emphasis on facilitative strategies.* To heal bodily symptoms, Western medicine focuses on how to combat the disease, kill the bacteria, and cut out the defective body parts. In its traditional biomedical model, illness (including mental illness) is considered to be an evil object, a threat to life, and an enemy against which patients must fight in order to survive. Any sign of weakness that is found in the patient is considered to be a triumph for the disease.

Similarly, distinct *fight* and *flight* responses are common among people who face trauma: in coping with cancer, we have *fighting spirit* versus *fatalism* (Watson, Law, dos Santos, & Greer, 1994); in dealing with grief, we have *confrontation* versus *avoidance* (Stroebe & Schut, 2001b). However, the use of the fight-or-flight dichotomy in coping research can be counterproductive, especially if it is based on the assumption that the former is adaptive and the latter is not. In Chinese philosophy, such an exclusivity of coping responses is unnecessary. From a traditional Chinese etiological point of view, disease is the manifestation of the patient's inner disharmony of energies. To heal is to strengthen the patient's entire bodily system by restoring the balance between different elements (internal organs) and systems (physical, psychosocial, and spiritual). A recent study shows that Chinese cancer patients use both *fight* and *flight* responses at the same time to cope with the disease (Ho, Fung, Chan, Watson, & Tsui, 2003). By surrendering themselves to the hands of fate, cancer patients gain a renewed sense of peacefulness while still doing what they can to live with the disease. In the realm of grief work research, there is still a lack of evidence that supports the hypothesis that avoiding one's grief is a less effective strategy than confronting it (Stroebe, 2001).

In social work practice, this warrior approach is also not uncommon. When dealing with the grief or fear that is commonly exhibited by people experiencing trauma, the *fight* against the irrational thinking of the client is often pictured as the ultimate battle that defines the outcome of the therapy. Nevertheless, although powerful in disputing maladaptive thinking (killing the bacteria), confrontational strategies (e.g., rational emotive therapy, Ellis, 1976) stop short at providing a nurturing environment in which the client can recuperate and grow (restoring balance and harmony). The SMART intervention does not ask clients to fight against their own belief system; instead, it fully acknowledges the need of the embattled client to retreat. Restoring clients' mental strength has a higher priority over using it to fight dysfunctional thinking, and this is done by meditation, healing rituals, social support, and philosophical teachings on pain and suffering (Chan, Ho, & Chow, 2001). The use of facilitative strategies rests on the assumption that healing comes from within (Saleebey, 1999).

> *Mrs. A, a middle-aged woman with breast cancer, joined our group for cancer patients two years ago. As a Buddhist, she learnt to be at peace with her cancer instead of fighting it all the time. Mrs. A wrote the following letter to her cancer, "My Dear Cancer, you shocked me. You ruined my plans and peace of mind . . . On the other hand, you reminded me of my mortality. My husband and children have become more caring and willing to express their love for me. My friends and relatives are also extremely helpful and shared with me how much I meant to them . . . Now that I have overcome the shock, I realize that you are actually part of me. You grew out of my cells. Thus, I have given you life and bring you to this world. You are like my children. No matter if my children are obedient or unruly, whether they do well in school or not, I accept them as they are . . . I accept you. As a part of me, I am at peace with you."*

*Promotion of dynamic coping.* In the Traditional Chinese Medicine paradigm, health and well-being result from a harmonious flow of "*qi*" (life energy) within the internal milieu of the person, and between the person and the external environment (Chan et al., 2001). Fixing our gaze on isolated symptoms and on external stressors is not necessarily the most effective way to heal (Tsuei, 1992; Yin, Zhang, Zhang, Zhang, & Meng, 1994). Neither is it desirable that clients who walk out from an intervention engage in only a single coping strategy, be it fight or flight. In the study of bereavement coping, Stroebe and Schut (2001a) observe a dynamic process of recovery, in which a bereaved person oscillates between internal preoccupation with grief (loss orientation) and external engagement with the outer world (restoration orientation). The purpose of clinical intervention, in this sense, is to remove obstacles to the cyclic flow of healing by encouraging clients to create and re-create their own coping strategies along the process.

## COMPONENTS OF SMART INTERVENTION

The SMART intervention incorporates activities that address the need for new sources of strength and meaning for our distressed clients.

The following describes the three aspects of intervention separately, but in practice these components are actually intertwined and integrated.

*Exploring alternative meanings through spiritual teaching.* The search for new meanings in life and a sense of peace is the essence of spirituality. In a religiously diverse world, we approach spirituality in a non-religious and generic way. "Why me?" "What is the meaning of this suffering?" "Why do bad things happen to good people?" These are the most common questions people ask during trauma or adversity. While not prescribing a particular principle of living, the following traditional Eastern spiritual teachings may serve to introduce new perspectives to clients.

1. Suffering–The Buddhist sees suffering as a necessary path to awakening. According to Buddhist teachings, there are eight types of suffering that are borne by mankind: birth, old age, sickness, death, being separated from loved ones, meeting people one hates, not getting what one wants, and sufferings caused by the senses of the body and the mind. Whereas the first four sufferings are products of nature's forces, the last four are borne out of attachment and expectations. Seeing suffering as inevitable to human existence can be a normalizing and calming process. To move out of suffering, one has to give up material and non-material attachments as well as to abandon unrealistic expectations.

2. Unpredictability–Daoist teaching places high value on the ever-changing reality of life and nature (*Dao*). As its founder Lao-zi described, "it is suffering that gives way to bliss; it is in bliss that suffering reveals" (Lao-zi, 6th century B.C.). To appreciate the unpredictability of life is to let go of intense emotional attachment to people and the material world. Accepting whatever comes in life, one can attain a state of being carefree.

3. Karma–The idea of karma can be seen as a primitive form of token economy. One major departure from the modern idea is that the karma system includes a relational aspect. A good deed of a person can benefit his or her loved ones. Conversely, to various degrees everybody has a shared burden of bad karma committed by mankind. Learning that their decisions on their well-being have an effect on the loved ones, clients are more willing to take charge of their own life, and to commit to a virtuous lifestyle.

4. Perseverance–Confucianism places high values on personal ordeals and see them as a blessing in disguise. "When Heaven is about to confer a great responsibility on any man, it will exercise

his mind with suffering" (Mencius, 6th century B.C., annotated by Tu, 1978). Being humble and filial in the face of hardship is the prescribed approach to coping with adversity.

It should be noted that the discussion of foregoing values appears in almost every major religions in the world. Deciding the most suitable way to present them requires the consideration of the clients' cultural background.

*Building strengths through physical expression.* There are a plethora of physical techniques in the East that can lead to spiritual growth. Among these, meditation (a Buddhist breathing practice), *tai-chi* (a traditional Chinese sport, also known as *tai-ji*), *qi-gong* (a Daoist form of exercise that incorporates breathing and movement), and yoga (a Hindu exercise) have withstood the test of time and are still popular in the modern world. A common feature of these ancient practices is the emphasis on body-mind-spirit interconnectedness. Under this principle, attempts have been made to adapt or modify these practices to better serve people in modern times. For example, Kabat-Zinn and his colleagues have developed the mindfulness-based stress reduction programs based on Zen Buddhism and yoga (Kabat-Zinn et al., 1992). Participants benefit from these meditation techniques by learning how to move away from their daily cognitive preoccupation, and to become mindful of the total existence of the person in the present moment. Another example is *tai-chi*. Evidence is emerging that this exercise is beneficial to both physical and mental health (Jin, 1992; Sandlund & Norlander, 2000). The *tai-chi* movements promote a disciplined approach to a frugal lifestyle, a healthy diet, and active physical labour. Physical benefits aside, the exercises of *tai-chi* and yoga can boost mental strength by reinforcing attention to bodily sensations and the endurance of pain.

Although it is not possible to teach *tai-chi* or yoga in a time-limited social work intervention, the first author extracted and simplified a set of movements such as body stretching and hand rubbing. Packaged as One-Second Techniques, these simple practices can be inserted into an intervention session (Chan, 2001). Being beneficial to health, these health-promotion practices also serve to distract clients from stress, and help them to regain a sense of control over their conditions as they can now take proactive measures to improve their total well-being.

*Consolidating new meanings and strengths through psycho-education.* To consolidate the newly acquired meanings and strengths, and to nurture those that already exist, we work on the cognitive, emotional and social well-being of clients to promote growth and transformation. The

SMART intervention addresses these aspects through the following strategies:

1. *Emphasizing growth through pain.* Instead of focusing on the loss that is brought on by crisis and trauma, personal strengths and gains are explored throughout the sessions. Although caution must be exercised to ensure that clients do not feel coerced or alienated, it is therapeutic for clients to be immersed in a positive environment in which they can briefly put aside the victim label that they are accustomed to and concentrate on the opportunities for growth and learning.

   *Mrs. B was diagnosed with SARS. She was put into an isolation ward in April 2003. Mrs. B was very scared, and used her mobile phone to communicate with the first author. During the discussion, Mrs. B was reminded to watch out for her personal growth and transformation, and to find ways to cope with her respiration difficulties. With this simple reminder to look out for growth, Mrs. B gained greater strength in withstanding her hospitalization and her days in intensive care.*

2. *Teaching the mind-body-spirit connection.* The relationship between spiritual well-being, mood, and body immunity is discussed with clients. When clients know they can improve their mood by taking care of their physical needs, and when they know how to do so by physical movements, breathing practices or massage, this sense of mastery can greatly boost their mental strength. Knowing that there can be things that one can do to help oneself is empowering.

   *Mr. C lost his job during SARS, as he worked in a hotel. He was depressed and at a loss as to what to do. As residents in Hong Kong were encouraged to go hiking and to engage in outdoor activities during the SARS period, he regained a sense of pride, confidence, and self-esteem by taking his daughter to country parks and teaching her exercises to strengthen her lungs. He regarded this period of unemployment as a special holiday that allowed him to spend time with his family, and viewed the loss of income a lesson in how to live a simple life.*

3. *Developing an appreciation of nature.* Being too self-absorbed with their own miseries, clients are often reluctant to turn their at-

tention to other areas of life. By appealing to the beauty of nature, clients are encouraged to appreciate their own life and appreciate people whom they love. We often start with the innocuous–birds in the sky, fishes in the ocean, and flora and fauna, and proceed to nature and the universe. We help clients to develop the habit of appreciating the small things in life, which slowly but steadily pulls clients away from their indulgence in pain.

*Mr. D, a teenager, developed SARS when he volunteered to help relocate an infected housing estate, Amoy Gardens (more than 200 residents of this housing estate were infected with SARS). He was very frustrated because he failed a public examination and lost his physical strength. Homebound, he learnt to pot plants at home. The new life of the small plants helped him to regain his appreciation of life and living.*

4. *Facilitating cognitive re-appraisal.* New perspectives can be developed through reflective discussions and sharing. Through the recall of significant life events, participants are reminded of their previous goals and dreams, their resilient experiences in facing other crises, and their past achievements in an attempt to foster a sense of confidence in their capacity of dealing with their present trauma. The positive psychology techniques of downward comparison, positive illusions, and learnt optimism are used to facilitate cognitive re-appraisal and the reconstruction of a new worldview (Taylor, Kemeny, Reed, Bower, & Gruenewald, 2000).
5. *Nourishing social support.* Effective interpersonal communication and a pleasant experience of networking can often nourish an individual's whole-person development, and especially enhances their resilience in difficult times. In a group environment, the participants will experience a sense of acceptance and connectedness with other group members. They are also encouraged to appreciate support from loved ones and to strengthen their social network with family members and friends. Mutual help among survivors with the same problems is an effective mechanism to sustain morale and the energy that is needed for change.
6. *Promoting the compassionate helper principle.* Clients are encouraged to learn from their traumatic experiences through being compassionate both to themselves and to other people. By sharing their knowledge and experiences in coping with traumatic events, clients are urged to consolidate their experiences and to become

sensitive to other people's needs. Being able to be helpful to others as peer counsellors can be very empowering. Selfless devotion to volunteering can move clients out of self-pity and into a path of recovery.

*Mr. E is a retired school principal who had a severe stroke soon after his retirement. He was in a coma for two months, and the attending physician described his prognosis as poor with a strong likelihood of permanent wheelchair dependency. With his strong willpower and resilience, he was able to walk again after a few months of active rehabilitation. He participated in mutual help activities for patients and became chair of the mutual help organization for stroke survivors after one year. He felt strongly that his meaning in life had changed, and his volunteering experiences had given him new abilities and strengths.*

We adapted these strategies in our intervention program through the use of writing (articles, lectures, books, and personal journals), expressive art (drawings, pictures, photos, and body movement) and multi-media materials (video, audiotapes, and CDs). Knowledge is delivered by showing videotapes of outstanding role models, and by distributing reading materials such as poems, research findings and personal testimonial. Throughout the intervention sessions, participants are encouraged to express their physical, mental and spiritual needs, as well as experiences of growth and transformation.

## IMPACT OF THE SMART INTERVENTION

The following is a summary of outcomes of SMART intervention with two groups of people (adolescents and people with chronic diseases) during SARS in Hong Kong, 2003 (Ng et al., 2004; Yau et al., 2004).

*Adolescents.* Adolescents in Hong Kong suffered from interruptions of normal academic and social life. Schools were suspended for a month for fear that the virus could spread in crowded places. Not only did students find it difficult to keep up with the learning schedule, but they were also excluded from the place where most of their social interaction and leisure activities took place. Without school as a location for social gathering, interpersonal relationships and social support were significantly hampered, and adolescents were at risk of becoming isolated and more prone to loneliness.

*People with chronic diseases.* People with a history of chronic disease faced a different kind of threat. The epidemiological profile of SARS cases in Hong Kong revealed an increased fatality rate in SARS-infected patients with chronic diseases (Drazen, 2003; Karlberg, Chong, & Lai, 2004; Peiris, Yuen, Osterhaus, & Stohr, 2003). Not only were they more susceptible to infection because of their health condition, but once infected, they also had a higher likelihood of death. Fear of infection (Society for Rehabilitation, 2003) and stigmatization (Hong Kong Mood Disorders Center, 2003b) were the two chief concerns among people with chronic diseases. As a result, many people in this group were in a state of fear and anxiety during the outbreak, and some did not dare to leave their homes months after the disappearance of SARS.

*Intervention.* To remove the adverse effects of SARS, the SMART intervention was applied to 244 Grade Eight students and 24 people with chronic diseases separately in the form of a one-day workshop. The program adopted a body-mind-spirit framework with a strong emphasis on a cognitive redefinition of SARS as *S*acrifice, *A*ppreciation, *R*eflection, and *S*upport. Participants were taught breathing exercises to strengthen their lungs, and skills to maintain a positive mood. Bitter tea and healthy snacks were served, and physical exercises, songs, fun, and positive experiences of growth through pain were shared. Through discussion and the sharing of personal reflections on the SARS experience, participants were more willing to accept the fact that life is not always within our control. SARS, natural disasters, accidents, crime, war, and trauma are all a part of life. What is more important is the reconstruction of meaning to reflect on what is most important in life. Participants were encouraged to attain a sense of mastery through letting go of control, and by so doing, regain control. The framework and rundown of the program are shown in Tables 1a and 1b, respectively.

*Outcome.* In an intervention program for adolescents at junior high school (Yau et al., 2004), it was found that the sense of social commitment, mastery of life, and learning and growth among the participants increased significantly after the intervention, and that their sense of social disintegration and loss of security decreased significantly. In a similar intervention for people with chronic diseases (Ng et al., 2004), participants reported a significant decrease in the Depression subscale scores of the Brief Symptom Inventory (BSI, Derogatis & Melisaratos, 1983), although changes in the Anxiety, Somatization, and Hostility

TABLE 1a. Framework of the SMART Intervention

|  | Foster awareness | Develop strength | Discover meaning |
|---|---|---|---|
| **Body** | Anxiety symptoms, lack of energy, appreciation of body, nurturing of body, importance of exercise | Physical exercise (e.g., movements, breathing exercises, tai-chi, acupressure), dietary advice (e.g., Chinese nutritional drinks, simple diet) | Acknowledge mind-body-spirit interconnectedness (e.g., somatization, optimism boosts immune system), physical exercises to foster total well-being |
| **Mind** | Fear, anxiety, anger, euphoria, frustrations, aggression, positive mood | Cognitive reappraisal relaxation and meditation, coping skills, learnt optimism, downward comparison | Recognize that issues of excess motions, both positive and negative emotions could be used in a constructive way to maintain harmony |
| **Spirit** | Lack of purpose, vulnerability of life, meaning in life, Eastern philosophy on perseverance | Life planning, goal setting, mindfulness, adoption of a Zen lifestyle to enhance inner strength and peace of mind, appreciation of life and nature | Appreciate the unpredictability of life, live for the moment, accept loss and mortality, selfless devotion to helping others, loving-kindness |

TABLE 1b. Structure of the SMART Intervention During the SARS Crisis

| Session One | Factual recapture:<br>- Brief recapture of the SARS pandemic<br>- Cognitive reappraisal: positive and negative impact of SARS<br><br>Revisiting symptoms:<br>- Discussion of impact on individuals and society<br>- Meditation on love for all<br><br>Coping with fear:<br>- Body-mind link: discussion of somatization<br>- Physical exercise: simple tai-chi, acupressure, massage<br>- Dietary advice: Traditional Chinese Medicine-derived health drinks to strengthen body<br>- Appreciation of life: Zen and Daoist teachings |
|---|---|
| **Session Two** | Emotional well-being:<br>- Chinese teachings: balance of emotional state<br>- Coping skills for excessive emotions<br><br>Creating meaning:<br>- Growth through pain, turning crisis into opportunity, finding creativity through trauma<br>- Life ahead, return to the basics, appreciate life and people<br>- Goal setting and action planning |

scores were not statistically significant. It was found that the drop in depression level was sustained in the intervention group but not in the control group at the one-month follow-up.

Despite the limitation of small sample size in the chronic patient intervention study, the preliminary data that is presented here shows that the SMART intervention can improve psychological states, and its effects can be maintained after one month. It is hypothesized that such an improvement was due to an increase of personal positive appraisal after the intervention, although further research is needed to confirm such a link.

## POTENTIAL CRITICISMS OF SMART INTERVENTION

As a novel attempt to incorporate the strengths perspective into trauma management, naturally there are reasonable suspicions about the SMART intervention.

*The SMART intervention is irrelevant in acute crises.* The primary goal of psychological debriefing is to alleviate distress through time-limited contact with a counselor. Although the promotion of growth and the building of strength in such settings might seem irrelevant at first glance, we found that the breathing and relaxation techniques activated self-confidence and inner strength, and promoted a sense of calmness and peace of mind within a relatively short period of time. Recent evidence indicates that although the alleviation of distress does not promote growth, the experience of growth does act to alleviate distress in the long run (e.g., Davis, Nolen Hoeksema, & Larson, 1998).

*The SMART intervention might alienate clients in distress.* When facing clients who are absorbed in turmoil and emotional distress, it is natural for individuals to contemplate whether it is appropriate to discuss growth and transformation with them. However, our clinical experience suggests otherwise. A supportive attitude and an invitation to grow through pain actually help to open a window of hope and optimism for clients who are engulfed by their sufferings. The delicate issue here is that instead of a Pollyanna denial or a direct confrontation of negative thoughts, a realistic and empathetic acknowledgement of the emotional pain of clients is required before any invitation to grow can be offered.

*The SMART intervention is a time-costly business.* Spiritual questing is known to be long and arduous. Pondering on the core values of the clients and making an appeal to their inner strengths is likely to be associated with the idea of intensive, long-term individual counseling that is far beyond the capacity of social workers with tight schedules. However, we believe that even in a single-session group, as we have demonstrated, social workers can work as catalysts and enablers of positive growth.

*The SMART intervention requires highly specialized experts.* Social workers may feel daunted by the prospect of investing time and effort in learning yet another set of intervention techniques. The model we are proposing here, however, is more of a set of guiding principles than of a list of step by step instructions. The creative use of techniques to work toward the right goal is more important than the acquisition of an arsenal of techniques without a target.

*The SMART intervention lacks empirical support.* One of the biggest limitations to strength-focused intervention is the lack of supporting empirical research. An early review of the research literature on using the strengths perspective for people with mental illnesses reveals a shortening of hospitalization time, improved social functioning, and a decrease in symptoms (Rapp, 1998). Although this early evidence cannot be translated into prescriptive recommendations, it is our hope that through rigorously designed experiments, future studies on strength-focused intervention may shed more light on its efficacy and applicability in various settings, including trauma management.

## CONCLUSION

This article argues for a holistic re-thinking of social work intervention in trauma management. Instead of being symptom-focused, we propose a strength-focused approach to help our clients to grow from suffering, to turn curses into blessings, and to promote creativity through pain. In addition to the enhancement of coping and problem solving abilities, social work intervention can expose clients to new horizons through the promotion of resilience and transformation through the reconstruction of meaning. Following traditional Eastern wisdom, we advocate an alternative to coping that is neither fight nor flight, and that encourages clients to accept and live through traumatic experiences with peace of mind, and to achieve a harmonious body-mind-spirit equilibrium. The use of integrative, multi-modal approaches, the emphasis on mind-body-spirit connectedness, and a dynamic view of coping form the backbone of the SMART intervention model. We believe that the proposed model can facilitate and catalyze such posttraumatic changes, although the emphasis on evidence-based practice in mainstream medicine and the social sciences requires a more methodologically sound research protocol (i.e., randomized control trial) and scientific indication. We therefore encourage social work practitioners and researchers to adapt the therapeutic elements of SMART to their respective cultural settings, and to carry out scientific research on the efficacy of SMART among different populations.

## REFERENCES

Bonanno, G. A. (2004). Loss, trauma, and human resilience: Have we underestimated the human capacity to thrive after extremely aversive events? *American Psychologist, 59*(1), 20-28.

Bonanno, G. A., Keltner, D., Holen, A., & Horowitz, M. J. (1995). When avoiding unpleasant emotions might not be such a bad thing: Verbal-autonomic response dissociation and midlife conjugal bereavement. *Journal of Personality and Social Psychology, 69*(5), 975-989.

Carlier, I. V. E. (2000). Critical incident stress debriefing. In A. Y. Shalev (Ed.), *International handbook of human response to trauma* (pp. 379-387). Dordrecht, Netherlands: Kluwer Academic Publishers.

Carlier, I. V. E., Voerman, A. E., & Gersons, B. P. R. (2000). The influence of occupational debriefing on post-traumatic stress symptomatology in traumatized police officers. *British Journal of Medical Psychology, 73*(1), 87-98.

Chan, C. L. W. (2001). *An Eastern Body-Mind-Spirit approach: A training manual with one-second techniques.* Hong Kong: University of Hong Kong.

Chan, C. L. W., Chan, Y., Law, W. F., Wong, F. L., & Yu, S. C. (1998). *Manual for emotional healing for divorced women.* University of Hong Kong, Hong Kong.

Chan, C. L. W., Chow, A., Au, T., Leung, P., Chau, P., Chang, F. et al. (1996). *Therapeutic groups in medical settings (Resource paper no. 25).* University of Hong Kong, Hong Kong.

Chan, C. L. W., Fan, F. W., & Gong, R. Y. (2003). *The Body-Mind-Spirit integrative health approach: Group counselling theory and application.* Beijing: Ethnic Publishing (in Chinese).

Chan, C. L. W., Ho, J., Ng, H. S., & Chau, M. (1996). *Quality of life for chronic patients: Report of the community rehabilitation network (Resource paper no. 27).* University of Hong Kong, Hong Kong.

Chan, C. L. W., Ho, P. S. Y., & Chow, E. (2001). A body-mind-spirit model in health: An Eastern approach. *Social Work in Health Care, 34*(3-4), 261-282.

Chan, C. L. W., & Rhind, N. (Eds.). (1997). *Social work intervention in health care,* Hong Kong: Hong Kong University Press.

Chapin, R., & Cox, E. O. (2001). Changing the paradigm: Strengths-based and empowerment-oriented social work with frail elders. *Journal of Gerontological Social Work, 36*(3-4), 165-179.

Chazin, R., Kaplan, S., & Terio, S. (2000). The strengths perspective in brief treatment with culturally diverse clients. *Crisis Intervention and Time Limited Treatment, 6*(1), 41-50.

Davis, C. G., Nolen Hoeksema, S., & Larson, J. (1998). Making sense of loss and benefiting from the experience: Two construals of meaning. *Journal of Personality and Social Psychology, 75*(2), 561-574.

Derogatis, L. R., & Melisaratos, N. (1983). The Brief Symptom Inventory: An introductory report. *Psychological Medicine, 13*(3), 595-605.

Drazen, J. M. (2003). SARS–Looking back over the first 100 days. *New England Journal of Medicine, 349*(4), 319-320.

Ellis, A. (1976). The rational-emotive view. *Journal of Contemporary Psychotherapy, 8*(1), 20-28.

Everly, G. S., Jr., & Boyle, S. H. (1999). Critical Incident Stress Debriefing (CISD): A meta-analysis. *International Journal of Emergency Mental Health, 1*(3), 165-168.

Fraser, J. S. (1998). A process view of crisis and crisis intervention: Critique and reformulation. *Crisis Intervention and Time Limited Treatment, 4*(2-3), 125-143.

Friedman, H. S. (2002). *Health Psychology* (2nd ed.). New Jersey: Pearson Education.

Graybeal, C. (2001). Strengths-based social work assessment: Transforming the dominant paradigm. *Families in Society, 82*(3), 233-242.

HKSAR Department of Health. (2003). *SARS Bulletin.* Retrieved March 25, 2004, from *http://www.info.gov.hk/dh/diseases/ap/eng/bulletin.htm*

Ho, S. M. Y., Fung, W. K., Chan, C. L. W., Watson, M., & Tsui, Y. K. Y. (2003). Psychometric properties of the Chinese version of the Mini-Mental Adjustment to Cancer (Mini-MAC) scale. *Psycho Oncology, 12*(6), 547-556.

Hong Kong Mood Disorders Center. (2003a, May 18). *Overview of mood disorders among Hong Kong people after SARS.* Retrieved March 25, 2004, from *http://www. hmdc.med.cuhk.edu.hk/report/report12.html*

Hong Kong Mood Disorders Center. (2003b, December 18). *Social and emotional disturbances among residents in Amoy Garden due to SARS.* Retrieved March 25, 2004, from *http://www.hmdc.med.cuhk.edu.hk/report/report16.html*

Hung, S. L., Kung, W. W., & Chan, C. L. W. (2003). Women coping with divorce in the unique sociocultural context of Hong Kong. *Journal of Family Social Work, 7*(3), 1-22.

Janoff Bulman, R. (1989). Assumptive worlds and the stress of traumatic events: Applications of the schema construct. *Social Cognition, 7*(2), 113-136.

Jin, P. (1992). Efficacy of Tai Chi, brisk walking, meditation, and reading in reducing mental and emotional stress. *Journal of Psychosomatic Research, 36*(4), 361-370.

Kabat-Zinn, J., Massion, A. O., Kristeller, J., Peterson, L. G., Fletcher, K. E., Pbert, L., et al. (1992). Effectiveness of a meditation-based stress reduction program in the treatment of anxiety disorders. *American Journal of Psychiatry, 149*(7), 936-943.

Karlberg, J., Chong, D. S., & Lai, W. Y. (2004). Do men have a higher case fatality rate of severe acute respiratory syndrome than women do? *American Journal of Epidemiology, 159*(3), 229-231.

Lamprecht, F., & Sack, M. (2002). Posttraumatic stress disorder revisited. *Psychosomatic Medicine, 64*(2), 222-237.

Lane, P. S. (1993). Critical incident stress debriefing for health care workers. *Omega: Journal of Death and Dying, 28*(4), 301-315.

Lao-zi. (6th century B.C.). *Tao Te Ching* (W. H. Chan, Trans.). Hong Kong: Commercial Press.

Lee, P. (1995). *An exploratory study of the effectiveness of relaxation techniques on rheumatoid arthritis patients.* Unpublished Master's dissertation, University of Hong Kong, Hong Kong.

Linley, P. A., & Joseph, S. (2004). Positive Change Following Trauma and Adversity: A Review. *Journal of Traumatic Stress, 17*(1), 11-21.

Man, W. K. (1996). *The empowering of Hong Kong Chinese families with a brain damaged member: Its investigation, measurement and intervention.* Unpublished Doctoral dissertation, University of Hong Kong, Hong Kong.

Miller, J. (2002). Affirming flames: Debriefing survivors of the World Trade Center attack. *Brief Treatment and Crisis Intervention, 2*(1), 85-94.

Mitchell, J. T., & Everly, G. S., Jr. (2000). Critical incident stress management and critical incident stress debriefings: Evolutions, effects and outcomes. In B. Raphael & J. P. Wilson (Eds.), *Psychological debriefing: Theory, practice and evidence* (pp. 71-90). New York, NY: Cambridge University Press.

Mitchell, J. T., Schiller, G., Eyler, V. A., & Everly, G. S., Jr. (1999). Community crisis intervention: The Coldenham tragedy revisited. *International Journal of Emergency Mental Health, 1*(4), 227-236.

Morgan, K. E., & White, P. R. (2003). The functions of art-making in CISD with children and youth. *International Journal of Emergency Mental Health, 5*(2), 61-76.

Moxley, D. P., & Washington, O. G. M. (2001). Strengths-based recovery practice in chemical dependency: A transpersonal perspective. *Families in Society, 82*(3), 251-262.

Neimeyer, R. A. (2000). *Lessons of loss: A guide to coping.* Memphis, Tennessee: Center for the Study of Loss and Transition.

Neimeyer, R. A. (2001). Reauthoring life narratives: Grief therapy as meaning reconstruction. *Israel Journal of Psychiatry and Related Sciences, 38*(3-4), 171-183.

Ng, S. M., Chan, T. H. Y., Chan, C. L. W., Lee, A., Yau, J. K. Y., Chan, C. H. Y. et al. (2004). *Group debriefing for persons with chronic diseases during the SARS pandemic: Strength-focused and Meaning-oriented Approach for Resilience and Transformation (SMART).* Unpublished manuscript.

O'Shea, B. (2001). Post-traumatic stress disorder: A review for the general psychiatrist. *International Journal of Psychiatry in Clinical Practice, 5*(1), 11-18.

Parkes, C. M. (1996). *Bereavement: Studies of grief in adult life* (3rd ed.). New York: International Universities.

Peiris, J. S., Yuen, K. Y., Osterhaus, A. D., & Stohr, K. (2003). The severe acute respiratory syndrome. *The New England Journal of Medicine, 349*(25), 2431-2441.

Peterson, A. L., Nicolas, M. G., McGraw, K., Englert, D., & Blackman, L. R. (2002). Psychological intervention with mortuary workers after the September 11 attack: The Dover Behavioral Health Consultant Model. *Military Medicine, 167*(Suppl9), 83-86.

Pollio, D. E., McDonald, S. M., & North, C. S. (1996). Combining a strengths-based approach and feminist theory in group work with persons "on the street." *Social Work with Groups, 19*(3-4), 5-20.

Rapp, C. A. (1998). *The strengths model: Case management with people suffering from severe and persistent mental illness.* New York: Oxford University Press.

Ray, O. (2004). How the mind hurts and heals the body. *American Psychologist January*, *59*(1), 29-40.

Robbins, A. (1998). Dance/movement and art therapies as primary expressions of the self. In A. Robbins (Ed.), *Therapeutic presence: Bridging expression and form* (pp. 261-270). London, England: Jessica Kingsley Publishers, Ltd.

Rose, S., Brewin, C. R., Andrews, B., & Kirk, M. (1999). A randomized controlled trial of individual psychological debriefing for victims of violent crime. *Psychological Medicine, 29*(4), 793-799.

Rowlands, A. (2001). Ability or disability? Strengths-based practice in the area of traumatic brain injury. *Families in Society, 82*(3), 273-286.

Russell, J. A., & Yik, M. S. M. (1996). Emotion among the Chinese. In M. H. Bond (Ed.), *The handbook of Chinese psychology* (pp. 166-188). London: Oxford University Press.

Russo, R. J. (1999). Applying a strengths-based approach in working with people with developmental disabilities and their families. *Families in Society, 80*(1), 25-33.

Saleebey, D. (1996). The strengths perspective in social work practice: Extensions and cautions. *Social Work, 41*(3), 296-305.

Saleebey, D. (1999). The Strengths Perspective: Principles and Practices. In B. R. Compton & B. Galaway (Eds.), *Social Work Processes* (6th ed.). CA: Brooks/Cole.

Sandlund, E. S., & Norlander, T. (2000). The effects of Tai Chi Chuan relaxation and exercise on stress responses and well-being: An overview of research. *International Journal of Stress Management, 7*(2), 139-149.

Schaefer, J. A., & Moos, R. H. (1998). The context for posttraumatic growth: Life crises, individual and social resources and coping. In R. G. Tedeschi, C. L. Park & L. G. Calhoun (Eds.), *Posttraumatic growth: Positive changes in the aftermath of crises* (pp. 99-125). Mahwah, NJ: Erlbaum.

Schaefer, J. A., & Moos, R. H. (2001). Bereavement experiences and personal growth. In M. S. Stroebe, R. O. Hansson, W. Stroebe & H. Schut (Eds.), *Handbook of bereavement research: Consequences, coping, and care* (pp. 145- 167). Washington, DC: American Psychological Association.

Schlenger, W. E., Caddell, J. M., Ebert, L., Jordan, B. K., Rourke, K. M., Wilson, D. et al. (2002). Psychological reactions to terrorist attacks: Findings from the National Study of Americans Reactions to September 11. *JAMA: Journal of the American Medical Association, 288*(5), 581-588.

Schneider, J. M. (1994). *Finding my way: Healing and transformation through loss and grief.* Colfax, WI: Seasons Press.

Schuster, M. A., Stein, B. D., Jaycox, L. H., Collins, R. L., Marshall, G. N., Elliott, M. N. et al. (2001). A national survey of stress reactions after the September 11, 2001, terrorist attacks. *New England Journal of Medicine, 345*(20), 1507-1512.

Sewell, J. D. (1993). Traumatic stress of multiple murder investigations. *Journal of Traumatic Stress, 6*(1), 103-118.

Society for Rehabilitation. (2003). *Survey report of the chronic patients' views of SARS.* Hong Kong: Society for Rehabilitation.

Stoll, B., & Edwards, L. A. (2002). Critical incident stress management with inmates: An atypical application. *International Journal of Emergency Mental Health, 3*(4), 245-247.

Stroebe, M. (2001). Gender differences in adjustment to bereavement: An empirical and theoretical review. *Review of General Psychology, 5*(1), 62-83.

Stroebe, M., & Schut, H. (2001a). Meaning making in the dual process model of coping with bereavement. In R. A. Neimeyer (Ed.), *Meaning reconstruction & the experience of loss* (pp. 55-73). Washington, DC: American Psychological Association.

Stroebe, M., & Schut, H. (2001b). Models of coping with bereavement: A review. In M. S. Stroebe (Ed.), *Handbook of bereavement research: Consequences, coping, and care* (pp. 375-403). Washington, DC: American Psychological Association.

Stroebe, M., Stroebe, W., Schut, H., Zech, E., & van den Bout, J. (2002). Does disclosure of emotions facilitate recovery from bereavement? Evidence from two prospective studies. *Journal of Consulting and Clinical Psychology, 70*(1), 169-178.

Sullivan, W. P., & Fisher, B. J. (1994). Intervening for success: Strengths-based case management and successful aging. *Journal of Gerontological Social Work, 22*(1-2), 61-74.

Taylor, S. E., Kemeny, M. E., Reed, G. M., Bower, J. E., & Gruenewald, T. L. (2000). Psychological resources, positive illusions, and health. *American Psychologist, 55*(1), 99-109.

Tedeschi, R. G., & Calhoun, L. G. (1995). *Trauma and transformation: Growing in the aftermath of suffering.* Thousand Oaks, CA: Sage Publications.

Thornton, A. A. (2002). Perceiving benefits in the cancer experience. *Journal of Clinical Psychology in Medical Settings, 9*(2), 153-165.

Tomich, P. L., & Helgeson, V. S. (2002). Five years later: A cross-sectional comparison of breast cancer survivors with healthy women. *Psycho Oncology, 11*(2), 154-169.

Tsai, J. L., & Levenson, R. W. (1997). Cultural influences of emotional responding: Chinese American and European American dating couples during interpersonal conflict. *Journal of Cross Cultural Psychology, 28*(5), 600-625.

Tsuei, W. (1992). *Roots of Chinese culture and medicine.* Java: Pelanduk Publications.

Tu, W. M. (1978). *Humanity and self-cultivation: Essays in Confucian thought.* Lancaster: Miller Publisher.

van Emmerik, A. A. P., Kamphuis, J. H., Hulsbosch, A. M., & Emmelkamp, P. M. G. (2002). Single session debriefing after psychological trauma: A meta-analysis. *Lancet, 360*(9335), 766-771.

Vickberg, S. M. J., Duhamel, K. N., Smith, M. Y., Manne, S. L., Winkel, G., Papadopoulos, E. B. et al. (2001). Global meaning and psychological adjustment among survivors of bone marrow transplant. *Psycho Oncology, 10*(1), 29-39.

Walker, J. P., & Lee, R. E. (1998). Uncovering strengths of children of alcoholic parents. *Contemporary Family Therapy: An International Journal, 20*(4), 521-538.

Watson, M., Law, M., dos Santos, M., & Greer, S. (1994). The Mini-MAC: Further development of the Mental Adjustment to Cancer scale. *Journal of Psychosocial Oncology, 12*(3), 33-46.

Wolfsdorf, B. A., & Zlotnick, C. (2001). Affect management in group therapy for women with posttraumatic stress disorder and histories of childhood sexual abuse. *Journal of Clinical Psychology, 57*(2), 169-181.

World Health Organization. (2003). *Severe acute respiratory syndrome (SARS): Status of the outbreak and lessons for the immediate future.* Retrieved March 25, 2004, from *http://www.who.int/csr/media/sars_wha.pdf*

Yau, J. K. Y., Chan, C. L. W., Lee, A., Chan, C. H. Y., Ng, S. M., Chan, A. et al. (2004). *Growth through SARS: Effectiveness of an intervention to build strength in adolescents in Hong Kong.* Paper presented at the Fourth International Conference in Social Work on Health and Mental Health, Quebec, Canada.

Yin, H. H., Zhang, B. L., Zhang, C. Y., Zhang, S. C., & Meng, S. M. (Eds.). (1994). *Foundations of Chinese medicine.* Shanghai: Shanghai Scientific.

Zebrack, B. (2000). Quality of life of long-term survivors of leukemia and lymphoma. *Journal of Psychosocial Oncology, 18*(4), 39-59.

# Extended Outpatient Civil Commitment and Treatment Utilization

### Steven P. Segal, PhD
### Philip Burgess, PhD

**SUMMARY.** *Objective*: This study considers four hypotheses regarding the impact of extended involuntary outpatient commitment orders on services utilization.

*Method*: All Victorian Psychiatric Case Register (VPCR) patients who had extended (180+ day) outpatient commitment orders in the nine year study period and a matched treatment compliant comparison group with extended periods of outpatient care (N = 1182), both with at least two years of post-episode experience, were evaluated. Pre/post episode utilization was compared via paired t tests with individuals as their own controls. Logistic and OLS regression as well as repeated measures ANOVA via the GLM SPSS program and post hoc t tests were used to evaluate between group and across time differences.

*Results*: Extended episodes of care for both groups were associated

Steven P. Segal is Professor and Director, Mental Health and Social Welfare Research Group, School of Social Welfare, University of California, Berkeley, Berkeley, CA 94720-7400. Philip Burgess is Professor, The University of Queensland, Mental Health Services Research, Queensland Centre for Mental Health Research, The Park–Centre for Mental Health, Wacol, Queensland, Australia.

Presented as the keynote address at The Ninth Doris Siegel Memorial Colloquium, International Social Health Care: Policy Program and Studies, held at the Mount Sinai Medical Center, New York, NY, May 20, 2004.

[Haworth co-indexing entry note]: "Extended Outpatient Civil Commitment and Treatment Utilization." Segal, Steven P., and Philip Burgess. Co-published simultaneously in *Social Work in Health Care* (The Haworth Press, Inc.) Vol. 43, No. 2/3, 2006, pp. 37-51; and: *International Social Health Care Policy, Programs, and Studies* (ed: Gary Rosenberg, and Andrew Weissman) The Haworth Press, Inc., 2006, pp. 37-51. Single or multiple copies of this article are available for a fee from The Haworth Document Delivery Service [1-800-HAWORTH, 9:00 a.m. - 5:00 p.m. (EST). E-mail address: docdelivery@haworthpress.com].

Available online at http://swhc.haworthpress.com
© 2006 by The Haworth Press, Inc. All rights reserved.
doi:10.1300/J010v43n02_04

with reduced use of hospitalization and increases in outpatient services. Extended orders did not promote voluntary participation in the post-period. Outpatient services during the extended episode for those on orders were raised to the level experienced by the treatment compliant comparison group and maintained at that level via subsequent renewal of orders throughout the patients' careers. OLS regression results indicate that approximately six community care service days were required for those on orders to achieve a one-day reduction in hospital utilization following the extended episode.

*Conclusion*: Outpatient commitment for those on extended orders in the Victorian context enables a level of community-based services provision, unexpected in the absence of this delivery system, which provides an alternative to hospitalization. *[Article copies available for a fee from The Haworth Document Delivery Service: 1-800-HAWORTH. E-mail address: <docdelivery@haworthpress.com> Website: <http://www.HaworthPress.com> © 2006 by The Haworth Press, Inc. All rights reserved.]*

**KEYWORDS.** Outpatient commitment, Victorian Psychiatric Case Register (VPCR), OLS regression, mental health

Involuntary outpatient commitment provisions are explicitly written into mental health laws in Australia, the United Kingdom, New Zealand, and 41 states and the District of Columbia in the United States (1-5). Though varying in their provisions, outpatient commitment orders require individuals (refusing care and believed potentially dangerous/gravely disabled due to a mental disorder) to accept community treatment or hospital release conditioned on treatment compliance (6). Such compliance may extend to requiring people to live in a particular apartment, take prescribed medications, attend counseling sessions, and abstain from substance utilization (1). Patients who do not comply with the treatment regimen in most jurisdictions may be admitted to a psychiatric hospital for involuntary care. In effect, the patient's status becomes one of conditional discharge from a psychiatric hospital whether or not they have been in the hospital (in some jurisdictions, orders may be issued without taking the individual to the hospital). This study looks at nine years of experience with the use of outpatient commitment in Victoria, Australia (see Table 1). It considers the claimed effectiveness of extended orders–outpatient commitments lasting longer than 180 days (3,4,7)–and moves beyond existing research by considering the complete patient careers of those put on orders and a matched treatment compliant comparison sample.

Outpatient commitment research has produced mixed results. Two major clinical trials in New York and North Carolina randomized small groups of patients (142 and 252 respectively) with mixed diagnoses at various points in their treatment careers to outpatient commitment and no outpatient commitment conditions and followed them for a year (3,8,9). Both studies failed to find significant differences between the randomized groups on any behavioral variables. In a secondary analysis, sacrificing the randomized component of the study, the North Carolina group found less hospital utilization among extended outpatient commitment patients (those with 180+ days on orders during the follow-up year). Four other studies, without comparison samples, are often cited as evidence that outpatient commitment reduces hospital admissions and the duration of hospital stays (10-13). Despite the failure

TABLE 1. Victoria's Outpatient Commitment: Community Treatment Orders

Outpatient commitment orders require individuals to accept outpatient treatment or hospital release conditioned on treatment compliance.

**Victoria's Eligibility Criteria: All of the following must obtain,**
- The person appears to be mentally ill; and,
- Their illness requires immediate treatment that can be obtained . . .
- For health or safety (whether to prevent a deterioration in physical or mental condition or otherwise) or for community protection; and,
- The person has refused treatment or is unable to consent to necessary treatment; and,
- No less restrictive option is available.

**How is outpatient commitment implemented in Victoria?**
- An authorised psychiatrist makes the Order (s.14 (1)) and the authorised psychiatrist or their delegate must monitor the treatment (s.14 (2)(a)).
- Patients may be placed on orders following hospital discharge or directly from the community.
- The Order can be extended indefinitely (s.14 (7)).
- The Order can be revoked by an authorised psychiatrist for non-compliance (s.14 (4)(b)).
- Patients whose treatment orders are revoked may be apprehended by the police and taken to an inpatient facility (s.14 (4A)).
- Entry to hospital occurs with somewhat less involved procedural safeguards than that of a direct admission. It is in effect a return from conditional leave.

**Patient Obligations?**
- Compliance with the order extends to requiring people to live in a particular apartment, take prescribed medications, and attend counseling sessions.

**What type of oversight is required?**
- Mental health review board hearing within eight weeks.
- Mental health review board review within 12 months.
- Review hearing on request by Mental Health Review Board (psychiatrist, attorney, mental health board staffers).

of the controlled trials to show differences attributable to outpatient commitment in the randomized group comparisons, the positive findings from the non-controlled studies and the extended outpatient commitment strategy of the North Carolina group, lead Applebaum (5), in an evaluation of the preponderance of evidence on such orders, to indicate that ". . . the weight of the evidence and clinical experience now favor efforts to implement reasonable schemes of outpatient commitment . . ." (p. 350). Following on the claims of the effectiveness of extended orders, advocates have come to see the extended period of such commitment as one such reasonable scheme (14). Given a need to replicate such findings, and a concern about the generalizability of the North Carolina results, further investigation of outpatient commitment and particularly its most promising scheme–180+ day extended orders–seems warranted.

In Victoria, Australia, the public mental health system covers 4.7 million inhabitants mandating a prescribed strategy of care emphasizing the desirability of community over inpatient treatment and care in the "least restrictive environment" (16-18). Since 1986 Victoria has relied on both the extensive use of outpatient commitment (to insure participation in prescribed care by patients believed unable to voluntarily accept needed treatment) and the aggressive and comprehensive outreach treatment approach employed in the Program In Assertive Community Treatment Model (PACT) (17). Mental health workers are expected to be in contact with the patient with a frequency dictated by the patient's condition and need for treatment. Given extended observation of different treatment teams (i.e., participation in home visits, counseling sessions, regular staff meetings involving the passing of care from one outpatient team shift to another, staffings involving extensive discussions of how, why and when an outpatient commitment should be employed, and watching several decisions to authorize such an order), it would appear that orders are initiated when team members cannot engage the patient in the services deemed necessary to ensure effective care–e.g., the patient, continuing to evidence disturbed behavior, does not attend counseling sessions or is absent when the team member visits so medication compliance cannot be adequately monitored. The objective of issuing orders is to prevent hospitalization by re-enabling contact with the patient with a frequency the team believes is necessary to insure compliance with prescribed treatment. Outpatient commitment can therefore be considered a successful alternative to hospitalization if it brings the level of service contact to that indicative of compliance with prescribed treatment.

Given previous research and the Victorian treatment objectives, the following four hypotheses are evaluated herein:

1. Extended outpatient commitment allows for relatively less use of inpatient treatment and will be accompanied by an increase in community care utilization (3).
2. Compliance post orders will be reflected in increases in voluntary care utilization (15).
3. Community care will substitute for inpatient care (16-18).
4. Outpatient commitment will enable the level of service provision to approximate that observed in a treatment compliant group.

## METHODS

### Sample

This retrospective study compares the service utilization of individuals placed on extended outpatient commitments, with a comparison group not placed on orders that experienced a psychiatric hospitalization and a voluntary extended period of community treatment, a treatment compliant sample. To the extent possible the groups are matched on variables influencing the probability of experiencing inpatient care episodes (19)–i.e., diagnosis, and gender and age (within 5 years). While the match is identical on diagnosis, it was not perfect on the latter two variables though all possibilities were exhausted.

The Victorian Psychiatric Case Register (VPCR) provides a record of all clinical contacts and their character occurring within the State. With approval of their ethics committee, the Victorian Department of Human Services approved our access to the register data. All patients having ever experienced an outpatient commitment between 12/11/90 and 30/6/00 (a period when in- and outpatient mental health service utilization and outpatient commitment could be reliably mapped using the VPCR) were identified along with a matched comparison sample (N = 7,826 pairs). In order to insure that we had information on the patient's entire pre-episode career and adequate post-episode follow-up (two years), we selected only those pairs (N = 2073 pairs) whose first contacts with the mental health system were on or later than 12/11/90 and who had first community care episode end dates prior to 30/6/98. Of these pairs, 1794 had complete outpatient commitment information–i.e., 86.5% of the sample; 591 pairs included both a patient with a 180+

day order and a matched comparison group member with a 180+ day community care episode (other pairs had patients with orders of shorter duration or no matched comparison with an extended care episode). The 591 pairs (N = 1182) constituted our evaluation sample.

## Units of Analysis

In documenting the treatment career experience, all treatment contacts were organized into episodes of care: each hospitalization (from day of admission to day of discharge) was considered a separate inpatient episode; each continuous period of community provision without a break in service $\geq$ 90 days, a community care episode (20). A service break followed by re-initiation of care was considered the start of a new community care episode. All occasions of community service are reported as community treatment days; multiple occasions of community service on the same day count as one community treatment day.

We consider the legal conditions under which treatment contacts occurred, reporting statistics separately for voluntary, involuntary, and combined total service utilization. Comparisons are based on yearly numbers of inpatient hospitalizations, hospital days, and/or community treatment days, thus adjusting for the period that the patient is at known risk for hospitalization or community service. A patient's career risk period is the date of first system contact to ninety days following the last system contact. If a patient left the area or died, this information can only be known by a ninety-day lapse in contact. Risk prior to the initial extended episode is measured from the patient's first date of system contact to the start date of the extended episode. Rates per year never reflect more treatment experiences than the patient actually had.

## Analyses (Employing the SPSS Statistical Package (21))

*Hypotheses 1 and 2: Reduced use of hospital and increased post-period voluntary compliance.* Using paired t tests, patients were considered within groups as their own comparisons. Patient experiences before the start of their first 180+ day episode were compared to their experiences after episodes' end. We assumed that the "before" experience would be significantly altered in the post-episode period and that the post-episode period experience would demonstrate whether treatment compliance could be voluntarily maintained (18).

*Hypothesis 3: Substitution of community care for inpatient.* Logistic and OLS Multiple Regression analyses were completed to respectively

evaluate whether the interaction effect of extended outpatient commitment and the receipt of community care significantly contributed to
avoiding post-period hospitalization or reducing post-period inpatient
days. Three groups of predictors were included in each model: 180+ day
episode duration, and duration of the follow up period, as controls for
exposure; age, gender, never married, under 65 and living on pension,
as previously demonstrated independent influences on hospital utilization; inpatient utilization per year prior to the 1st 180+ day episode, as a
severity adjustment (22); and, community care days per year following
the start of the episode, group membership and the interaction of the
later two variables, the interventions.

*Hypothesis 4: Outpatient commitment will enable service contact to
approximate that observed in a treatment compliant group.* In making
between group and across time comparisons we used the GLM program
to consider overall differences in utilization of community services and
to address two post hoc comparisons: community treatment utilization
differences between groups during the extended episode and during vs.
post-episode for the group on orders.

## RESULTS

The sample's ICD-9CM primary diagnoses are: schizophrenia (N =
1050, 88.8%), major affective disorder (N = 60, 5.1%), and other conditions (N = 72, 6.1%). Though matched on diagnosis, age within five
years, and gender there were differences between groups on the latter two
variables (see Table 2). While no statistical differences were found in the
duration of the follow up periods for the two groups, the time of their involvement with the system prior to their initial extended episode, the duration of that episode, their career hospitalizations, and the extent of
community involvement prior to each of their admissions, did differ. The
first finding allows us to make post-period between group comparisons
with greater confidence regarding intervention exposure effect compara-
bility; the latter differences are into taken account in the statistical models
and by making our comparisons based on yearly utilization. Further, the
treatment compliant status of the comparison group seems to be validated
in that this group voluntarily participated in community treatment for an
average period of 392 days. While it is difficult to define treatment compliance, such participation among those meeting hospitalization criteria
seems a reasonable test.

TABLE 2. Demographics and Design Relevant Patient Career Statistics

| Characteristic | Comparison | Outpatient Commitment | Total |
|---|---|---|---|
| | N (%)/M (sd) | N (%)/M (sd) | N (%)/t,df,p |
| **Total Sample** | 591  (50%) | 591  (50%) | 1182  (100%) |
| **Gender** | | | |
| Male | 415 (70.2%) | 350 (59.2%) | 765  (64.7%) |
| Female | 176 (29.8%) | 241 (40.8%) | 417 (35.3%) |
| | | | |
| **Age at First Date** | 26.59 (11.10) | 34.01 (16.01) | 30.31 (14.26) |
| | | | |
| **Marital Status** | | | |
| Divorced | 32  (5.4%) | 49  (8.3%) | 81  (6.9%) |
| Defacto Cohabiting Partner | 28  (4.7%) | 27  (4.6%) | 55  (4.7%) |
| Married (Legally) | 60 (10.2%) | 73 (12.4%) | 133 (11.3%) |
| Never Married | 422 (71.4%) | 339 (57.4%) | 761 (64.4%) |
| Separated | 33  (5.6%) | 59 (10.0%) | 92  (7.8%) |
| Widowed | 5  (0.8%) | 34  (5.8%) | 39  (3.3%) |
| Unknown | 11  (1.9%) | 10  (1.7%) | 21  (1.8%) |
| | | | |
| **Duration of 1st 180+ Day Episode** | 492 days (sd 382) | 391days (sd 214) | $t = 5.56$, df 590, $p < .000$ |
| **Duration of Follow-up Period** | 904 days (sd 742) | 841 days (sd 667) | $t = -1.57$, df = 590, $p = .115$ |
| **Days From 1st System Contact To 1st 180+ Day Episode** | 374 days (sd 526) | 685 days (sd 612) | $t = -9.81$, df = 590, $p < .000$ |
| **Average # of Times Community Involved Prior to Admission** | 2.52 (sd 1.94) | 4.36 (sd 3.51) | $t = -12.1$, df = 460, $p < .000$ |

*Hypotheses 1 and 2: Findings indicate a reduced use of hospital, an increase in post-period community care, but no increase in post-period voluntary compliance.* Table 3 shows that patients on orders were hospitalized on average 56.3 days per year before the extended episode and only 19.6 days per year after. Their number of community treatment days increased from 27.5 days per year to 41.1 days per year in the respective periods. The comparison sample was hospitalized on average 37.2 days per year before and only 10.4 days per year after. Their number of community treatment days increased from 13.3 days per year to18.8 days per year. The differences are significant at p < .000 as are all before and after comparisons in Table 3 with one noted exception. Increases in voluntary community treatment days were *not* significant for those on orders. For this group the increases were primarily in the involuntary community treatment day category. For the comparison group community treatment day increases were all in the voluntary category. (The few involuntary community contacts reflect involvement of community-based staff during an involuntary hospitalization to insure continuity of care; involvements decreased across periods due to actual reductions in involuntary hospitalizations.)

*Hypothesis 3: There was a significant substitution of outpatient care for inpatient care.* Table 4 shows the results of the logistic and OLS regressions predicting, respectively, post-period hospitalization and post-period utilization of inpatient days. The logistic model is significant (Chi Sq. 423.265, df 10 p < .000) and demonstrates that when all factors are taken into account each day of community treatment decreases the chance of hospitalization in the post-period for the outpatient commitment group by 3.2% over those in the comparison group. The OLS model is significant (AdjRsq = .101, F = 13.202, df = 10,1089, p < .000). It shows a significant outpatient commitment group by community care service days interaction (b = −.16, se .06, p < .004) such that for the outpatient commitment group (with all other covariates and demographics controlled) one community treatment day is associated with a .16 reduction in inpatient days per year during the period after the episode end; alternatively six community treatment days with a one (.96) day reduction in inpatient utilization.

*Hypothesis 4: Outpatient commitment enabled service contact to approximate that observed in a treatment compliant group.* The groups differed in their utilization of outpatient services across the three points in time (F = 106.51, p < .000) as did the subjects within groups (F = 297.22, p < .000). Of most importance, however, is the absence of significant differences between groups in their yearly community service utilization *during* the extended episode and between the *episode and post episode periods* for the group on orders (see Figure 1).

TABLE 3. Service Utilization Before, During, and After First 180 Day Episode (N = 591)

| Service Type | Outpatient Commitment Group | | | | | | Comparison Group | | | | | |
|---|---|---|---|---|---|---|---|---|---|---|---|---|
| | Before Start | | During | | After End | | Before Start | | During | | After End | |
| | Mean | SD | Mean | SD | Mean | SD | Mean | SD | Mean | SD | Mean | SD |
| **Hospitalization Inpatient Days** | | | | | | | | | | | | |
| Involuntary | 47.3 | 55.4 | NA | NA | 17.0 | 32.0 | 25.8 | 33.0 | NA | NA | 5.9 | 14.4 |
| Voluntary | 9.1 | 27.1 | NA | NA | 2.6 | 8.4 | 11.4 | 25.6 | NA | NA | 4.5 | 18.1 |
| Total | 56.3 | 82.5 | NA | NA | 19.6 | 40.4 | 37.2 | 58.6 | NA | NA | 10.4 | 32.5 |
| **Number of Admissions** | | | | | | | | | | | | |
| Involuntary | 1.3 | 0.9 | NA | NA | 0.6 | 0.8 | 0.9 | 0.7 | NA | NA | 0.4 | 0.7 |
| Voluntary | 0.3 | 0.6 | NA | NA | 0.1 | 0.4 | 0.5 | 0.8 | NA | NA | 0.3 | 0.5 |
| Total | 1.7 | 1.5 | NA | NA | 0.7 | 1.2 | 1.4 | 1.5 | NA | NA | 0.7 | 1.2 |
| **Average Length of Stay in Days** | | | | | | | | | | | | |
| Involuntary | 24.0 | 34.6 | NA | NA | 7.0 | 14.1 | 19.4 | 24.5 | NA | NA | 4.3 | 10.5 |
| Voluntary | 5.9 | 22.6 | NA | NA | 1.8 | 7.0 | 7.3 | 15.7 | NA | NA | 2.6 | 13.4 |
| **Community Care Days** | | | | | | | | | | | | |
| Voluntary | 18.3 | 22.2 | .2 | 3.8 | 19.9 | 26.5 | 11.7 | 17.4 | 41.8 | 24.7 | 18.1 | 22.3 |
| Involuntary | 9.2 | 17.9 | 42.3 | 32.7 | 21.2 | 34.4 | 1.5 | 2.9 | .5 | 4.1 | 0.7 | 2.4 |
| Totals | 27.5 | 40.2 | 42.8 | 32.3 | 41.1 | 61.0 | 13.3 | 20.2 | 42.0 | 24.6 | 18.8 | 24.7 |

## TABLE 4. Hospitalization and Inpatient Days Post Period Following 1st 180+ Day Community Episode

**A. Hospitalization in the Post Period Logistic Regression Model\***

Variables in the Equation\*\*

|  | B | S.E. | Wald | df | Sig. | Exp(B) |
|---|---|---|---|---|---|---|
| • GROUP = Outpatient Commitment v Comparison | .696 | .289 | 5.797 | 1 | .016 | 2.006 |
| • Community Service days per year after the start of the 1st 180+ Day Episode | .039 | .006 | 41.912 | 1 | .000 | 1.040 |
| • Interaction: Outpatient Commitment Group by Community Service Days After the Start of the 1st 180+ Day Episode | −.032 | .006 | 28.456 | 1 | .000 | .968 |

\*Dependent variable: Hospitalized in the post period (Chi Sq. 423.265, df 10 p < .000).

\*\*Predictor Variables in the Equation: Group, interaction of group by treatment days after the start of the 180+ episode, age, gender, never married, pension income, follow-up period duration, 1st 180+ period duration, inpatient days per year prior to the 1st 180+ episode, treatment days following the start of the 180+ episode. Only the main group and service effects, and the interaction effect are shown.

**B. Inpatient Days Per Year in the Post Period OLS Regression Model**

|  | Unstandardized Coefficients | | Standardized Coefficients | t | Sig. |
|---|---|---|---|---|---|
|  | B | Std. Error | Beta | | |
| (Constant) | −7.495 | 4.482 | | −1.672 | .095 |
| • Group: (Outpatient Commitment = 1, Comparison = 0) | 8.411 | 2.906 | .152 | 2.894 | .004 |
| • Community service days per year after the start of the 1st 180+ Day Episode | .223 | .054 | .519 | 4.124 | .000 |
| • Interaction of Outpatient Commitment Group by Community Service Days After the Start of 180 Day Episode | −.161 | .056 | −.424 | −2.893 | .004 |

\*Dependent variable: Total inpatient days per year after the end of the 1st 180 episode; R = .330, Rsq = .101, Adj. Rsq. = .101, F = 13.202, D.f. = 10,1089, p < .000.

\*\*Predictor Variables in the Equation: Group, interaction of group by treatment days after the start of the 180+ episode, age, gender, never married, pension income, follow-up period duration, 1st 180+ period duration, inpatient days per year prior to the 1st 180+ episode, treatment days following the start of the 180+ episode. Only the main group and service effects, and the interaction effect are shown.

FIGURE 1. Yearly Service Utilization Before, During, and After Episode

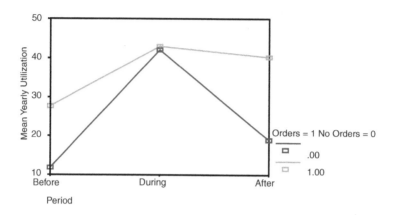

## *DISCUSSION*

Comparisons of the pre/post extended community care episode utilization experiences of both groups show reduced use of hospitalization, approximately a month per year per patient, and dramatic increases in
community services, approximately a third more service utilization than
in the pre-period. This is, however, only a partial support of the first hypothesis since proportionally the reductions and increases are similar for
both groups and might be attributed to deinstitutionalization policy in
Victoria or simple regression to the mean. Most important, however, with
respect to evaluating the utility of outpatient commitment, is that the
equivalent proportional increase in the community services for the group
on orders, and perhaps the proportional reduction in the hospitalization,
only arises because of the provision of ordered community care.

Outpatient commitment is a way of delivering services to a population that for one or another reason cannot or will not consistently accept
such service voluntarily. It would appear that the role of the outpatient
commitment *during* the extended episode is to raise the level of outpatient service to that provided to the treatment compliant comparison
sample. We observed no difference in the total amount of community
services used in both groups during the extended episode–the comparison group received them voluntarily, the committed group under orders.
Extended orders from their initiation represent a change in the way of

packaging services for a patient and the process is continued via renewals following the initial episode's end throughout the patient's career. Long-term service participation under orders does not presage a shift to voluntary participation.

Outpatient commitment provided an alternative to hospitalization during the episode when no hospitalization occurred as well as in the post-period. In the post-period our regression analyses demonstrate that *it is the combination of community services enabled by outpatient commitment that facilitate the reduction of hospital utilization in the population on extended orders.* In the outpatient commitment group this results in the substitution of approximately six outpatient community treatment days for each reduced inpatient day per year in the period after the end of the 1st extended episode. Thus, extended outpatient commitment enables community services to become an alternative to hospitalization, without it there would be limited service participation for the group on orders.

Neither extended outpatient commitment alone nor community services alone accounted for the reduced inpatient day use effect in the post-period—quite the opposite. As in other studies (1), both are associated with increased inpatient utilization because such services are frequently initiated around the crises preceding an inpatient care episode and accompany the transition from hospital back to community. We believe that the use of such findings to argue against the use of extended orders fails to appreciate the role of the outpatient commitment in community care efforts.

*Outpatient commitment is perhaps best conceived as a delivery mechanism rather than a treatment in and of itself.* It is probably only as good as the treatment that accompanies it. Given that the alternative to hospitalization effect is accomplished through the additional use of involuntary community care in the follow-up period, it is difficult for many to identify the involuntary commitment as a success. Yet, the patients on orders are complex cases whose services needs are probably more extensive than the treatment compliant matched controls at the outset (1). Witness that prior to each hospitalization the community involvement with the patients on orders is almost twice that of the comparison group.

Our findings speak only to the use of extended 180+ day episodes of care in combination with community services offered in Victoria, Australia. They do not address demonstrable psychosocial outcomes experienced by individuals participating in such treatment regimens. The results and conclusions reported herein might be considered stronger from an evidence standpoint had they been derived from comparisons of randomly assigned groups, yet the RCT vehicle would not have offered a nine-year representation of a population's real world experience. We did use a matched comparison design with patients acting as their own controls in the within and between group analyses. Moreover, though our findings apply only to the Australian context, it is notable that outpatient commitment has become a major issue in Western psychiatry and this study represents a report on the most extensive experience with its utilization.

This paper offers several new perspectives on outpatient commitment: It considers outpatient commitment as a delivery system. It focuses on the interaction of outpatient commitment with services provided and questions previous approaches that criticize the use of outpatient commitment on the basis of its associations with increased service utilization. In conclusion, *outpatient commitment for those on extended orders in the Victorian context enables a level of community-based services provision, unexpected in the absence of this delivery system, which provides an alternative to hospitalization.*

## REFERENCES

1. Preston NJ, Kisely S, Xiao J: Assessing the outcome of compulsory psychiatric treatment in the community: Epidemiological study in Western Australia. British Journal of Medicine 524:1244-1246, 2002

2. Torrey EF, Kaplan RJ: A national survey of the use of outpatient commitment. Psychiatric Services 46: 778-784, 1995

3. Swartz MS, Swanson JW, Hiday VA et al.: Can involuntary commitment reduce hospital recidivism? Findings from a randomized trial with severely mentally ill individuals. American Journal of Psychiatry 12: 1968-1974, 1999

4. Swartz MS, Swanson JW, Hiday VA et al.: A randomized controlled trial of outpatient civil commitment in North Carolina. Psychiatric Services 52(3): 325-329, 2001

5. Appelbaum P: Thinking carefully about outpatient commitment. Psychiatric Services 52(3): 347-351, 2001

6. Allen M, Smith VF: Opening Pandora's Box: The practical and legal dangers of involuntary outpatient commitment. Psychiatric Services 52(3): 342-347, 2001

7. Torrey EF, Zdanowicz MT: Outpatient commitment: What, why, and for whom. Psychiatric Services 52(3): 337-341, 2001

8. Policy Research Associates Final Report: Research Study of the New York City Involuntary Outpatient Commitment Pilot Program, (at Bellevue Hospital). Policy Research Associates (www.prainc.com/IOPT/opt toc.ht), 1998

9. Steadman HJ, Gounts K, Dennis D et al.: Assessing the New York City Involuntary Outpatient Commitment Pilot Program. Psychiatric Services 52(3): 330-337, 2001

10. Fernandez GA, Nygard S: Impact of involuntary outpatient commitment on the revolving door syndrome in North Carolina. Hospital and Community Psychiatry 41: 1001-1004, 1990

11. Zanni G, deVeau, L: Inpatient stays before and after outpatient commitment in Washington, DC Hospital and Community Psychiatry 37: 941-942, 1986

12. Munetz MR, Grande T, Kleist J et al.: The Effectiveness of Outpatient Civil Commitment. Psychiatric Services 47: 1251-1253, 1996

13. Rohland B: The role of outpatient commitment in the management of persons with schizophrenia. Iowa Consortium for Mental Health Services, Training, and Research, 1998

14. Torrey EF, Zdanowicz MT: Study shows that long-term assisted treatment reduces violence and hospital utilization. Catalyst 2(3): 1-2, 2000

15. Van Putten DA, Santiago JP, Bergen MR: Involuntary commitment in Arizona: A retrospective study. Hospital and Community Psychiatry 39:205-502, 1988

16. Commonwealth of Australia: National Mental Health Report 1996, Canberra, ACT: Commonwealth Department of Health and Family Services, 1998

17. Commonwealth of Australia: National Mental Health Report 1997. Canberra, ACT: Commonwealth Department of Health and Family Services, 1999

18. Mental Health Branch National Standards for Mental Health Services. Canberra, ACT: Commonwealth Department of Health and Family Services, 1997

19. Robins L, Regeir D (Eds.): Psychiatric Disorders in America: The Epidemiological Catchment Area Study. New York: The Free Press, 1991

20. Tansella M, Micciolo R, Biggeri A et al.: Episodes of care for first-ever psychiatric patients: A long term case-register evaluation in a mainly urban area. British Journal of Psychiatry 167, 220-227, 1995

21. SPSS for Windows, Release 11.0.1, 2001

22. Schinnar AP, Rothbard AB, Kanter R: Adding state counts of the severely and persistently mentally ill. Administration and Policy in Mental Health 19(1): 3-12, 1991

# From a Social Issue to Policy:
# Social Work's Advocacy for the Rights
# of Donor Conceived People
# to Genetic Origins Information
# in the United Kingdom

Elizabeth Wincott, CSW
Marilyn Crawshaw, MA, BSc(Soc), CQSW, DipAppSocStudies

**SUMMARY.** This paper outlines a 22 year campaign to introduce openness into the arena of donor conception in the UK. It identifies key aspects of the development of an advocacy based approach to such work and argues that social work values and principles can prove key to identifying structural inequalities which are not necessarily based in socio-economic disadvantage. Donor conceived people may find them-

Elizabeth Wincott resides in Oxford, United Kingdom. Marilyn Crawshaw is affiliated with Department of Social Policy and Social Work, University of York, York, England.

Address correspondence to: Marilyn Crawshaw, Department of Social Policy & Social Work, University of York, York, YO10 5DD, England (E-mail: mac7@york.ac.uk).

The authors would like to acknowledge the support of Progar members in the compilation of this paper and especially Eric Blyth.

This article is based on a paper given by Elizabeth Wincott at the Doris Siegel Colloquium in New York in 2004.

[Haworth co-indexing entry note]: "From a Social Issue to Policy: Social Work's Advocacy for the Rights of Donor Conceived People to Genetic Origins Information in the United Kingdom." Wincott, Elizabeth, and Marilyn Crawshaw. Co-published simultaneously in *Social Work in Health Care* (The Haworth Press, Inc.) Vol. 43, No. 2/3, 2006, pp. 53-72; and: *International Social Health Care Policy, Programs, and Studies* (ed: Gary Rosenberg, and Andrew Weissman) The Haworth Press, Inc., 2006, pp. 53-72. Single or multiple copies of this article are available for a fee from The Haworth Document Delivery Service [1-800-HAWORTH, 9:00 a.m. - 5:00 p.m. (EST). E-mail address: docdelivery@haworthpress.com].

Available online at http://swhc.haworthpress.com
© 2006 by The Haworth Press, Inc. All rights reserved.
doi:10.1300/J010v43n02_05

selves in families which enjoy material privilege but whose exposure to a legislative framework and dominant professional cultures within the treatment centres encourages secrecy around genetic origins. Social workers' experience of adoption and family work leads them to recognise the danger of such secrets within families. Turning such social issues into policy changes requires vision, strategic long term advocacy and partnership with those directly affected. *[Article copies available for a fee from The Haworth Document Delivery Service: 1-800-HAWORTH. E-mail address: <docdelivery@haworthpress.com> Website: <http://www.HaworthPress.com>* © 2006 by The Haworth Press, Inc. All rights reserved.]*

**KEYWORDS.** Advocacy, social work values, donor conception, secrecy in families

## BACKGROUND

Following the birth of the world's first so-called test tube baby, Louise Brown, in 1978, there was was a rapid growth in knowledge about, and development of, an ever expanding variety of techniques to assist reproduction. However, the clinics providing these services in the UK were largely private and unregulated except through an emerging voluntary system run by a voluntary licensing authority. The lack of a statutory regulation system on all aspects including gamete storage and donation, access, record keeping and new developments together with the lack of external accountability and scrutiny in this ethically challenging area of medical science led to the government setting up a Committee of Inquiry into Human Fertilisation and Embryology in 1982 to consider recent and potential developments in medicine and science related to human fertilisation and embryology; to consider what policies and safeguards should be applied, including consideration of the social, ethical and legal implications of these developments; and to make recommendations. It was chaired by Dame Mary Warnock, Mistress of Girton College Cambridge and a moral philosopher (Warnock, 1984).

Social work's professional body, the British Association of Social Workers (BASW), submitted evidence to the Committee through its Health and Handicap Advisory Panel and Sexuality Special Interest Group in March 1983.

The Warnock Committee reported in 1984 and recommended that legislation be brought forward to provide for statutory regulation. In doing so, it made a number of recommendations that had the potential to deeply affect family life and children's welfare. These included the recommendation that children conceived using donated gametes should not be afforded the right to receive information about the identity of their donor when they attained the age of majority. This was despite the passing of the Adoption Act of 1976 which had extended the rights of adopted people in England and Wales at the age of majority to disclosure of the identity of their birth parents, both retrospectively and prospectively.

Several initiatives within BASW were brought together to set up the Warnock Report Project Group in October 1984 to respond to the Committee's findings. The membership was drawn entirely from social workers and BASW staff with its focus underpinned by social work values, principles and practice. Of fundamental concern was the Warnock Committee recommendation that gamete donation should be anonymous which was felt to be contradictory to the rights (moral and human) and needs (social and psychological) of people to have access to their personal biographies.

Thus commenced BASW's lobby for the right of donor conceived people to have parity with adopted people–the only other group of people at that time whose families had come into being as a result of professional intervention and whose access to information about their genetic relationships was regulated by statute. When subsequent legislation to regulate surrogacy (the Surrogacy Arrangements Act 1985) opted for parity with adopted people with regard to accessing identifying information from age 18, donor conceived people were further marginalised and BASW made strong representation about the inconsistency and resulting discrimination.

This paper covers the 22-year period through to the lifting of anonymity and documents the campaign that was conducted through the social work professional association to advocate on behalf of people conceived and to-be conceived using donor assisted conception techniques. It describes the development of the campaign to include those directly affected as well as other professional groups; the attention to strategic planning; and the engagement with policy makers and opinion formers. It argues that social work has a central role to play in such work and that attention to social work values is as vital as ever in offering the vision for such work.

## THE INTRODUCTION OF LEGISLATION

In November 1987 the government published a White Paper on the framework for proposed legislation. BASW was invited to provide further input at this stage and also gave oral evidence to a Parliamentary Standing Committee in 1988.

In May 1988 two additional members–an academic social scientist and an experienced counsellor in an assisted conception clinic (and ex-social worker)–were co-opted. In October 1988 the name was formally changed from the Warnock Project Group to the Project Group on Assisted Reproduction (Progar) to avoid confusion with the Warnock Committee.

After the Human Fertilisation & Embryology Bill was published in 1989, Progar continued to lobby extensively around the rights of donor conceived people. However, although some changes were made in the drafting, the underlying policy of retaining the anonymity of donors remained.

The Human Fertilisation and Embryology Act was passed in 1990 and the Human Fertilisation and Embryology Authority (HFEA) set up as the regulatory body in August 1991. It was required to hold a database of the details of all live assisted conception births, including social details of donors and their medical history. From this a Register of Information was to be derived and donor conceived people were given the legal right at 18 to access information about whether they were on the Register (and hence donor conceived) or at 16 to discover whether they were related through donor conception to anyone that they intended to marry. Although Regulations to allow for the release of non-identifying information were not enacted until 2004, it was always anticipated that this would happen. A small section on the official form that is sent to the HFEA about each cycle of treatment is provided for donors to provide pen pictures of themselves and some, though not all, centres encourage the completion of this. However, a study of the information held was found to be patchy and inconsistent (Blyth & Hunt, 1998). Some of the pen portraits were treated so facetiously as potentially to cause distress to any offspring reading them.

The first people to reach 16 will do so in 2008. Between 1991 and April 2005, upwards of 24,000 donor conceived people were estimated to be born and were the only people in the UK for whom the state held identifying information on their genetic origins to which they were denied access.

## BUILDING THE CASE FOR LEGISLATIVE
## AND PRACTICE CHANGES

Following the introduction of the HFE Act, Progar determined to continue to lobby for change. It did so in a number of ways, paying careful attention to strategic planning within limited resources.

### Widening the Membership

During the 1990s Progar decided to widen its membership to include those directly affected and their families, other disciplines, and key social welfare organisations including:

- two donor conceived people, one a psychologist and one a lawyer
- a mother of donor conceived children who, together with her husband, had set up a UK wide network of parents of donor conceived children called DC Network
- a representative from the Association of Directors of Social Service, the body which represents all statutory social services in England and Wales
- a lawyer specialising in children's law and adoption
- a representative from the British Infertility Counselling Association (BICA)
- representatives of three major UK children's charities

At the same time as inviting the HFEA to attend as observers, an invitation was extended to (and accepted by) the UK Department of Health (DH) to attend, also with observer status.

This extended membership gave Progar links into wider networks thus enabling it to promote and influence wide-ranging and diverse debates. It also undoubtedly afforded it greater clout in its own campaigning and ensured greater coverage of its views in the media and amongst political and other influential figures. From time to time, invitations to meetings were extended to those whom Progar thought had the potential to be allies, not least to assist in discussion of strategy. The fact that such figures as Allan Levy QC, the leading children's barrister, David Hinchliffe, Chair of the Parliamentary Select Committee on Health and Baroness Mary Warnock herself accepted was an indication of Progar's growing stature. Indeed it was to Progar that Baroness Warnock indicated her change of mind about anonymity and agreed to share our platform in campaigning for change.

## *Use of the Media and Being in the Public Eye*

Increasingly, members developed a speaking profile in the professional and public media and were regularly sought out for public comment. Growing numbers of written contributions were valued in professional and academic journals and in the media. Members contributed regularly to national and international conferences. The foci of the debates that emerged were wide-ranging and there was active discussion within Progar both about its own standpoint and about the most strategically useful approach to take in different arenas. For example, the arguments were variously presented with a primary focus on the impact of secrecy on psychological well being, the primacy of children's rights over the rights of infertile adults to found a family, the impact of inadequate or inaccurate medical history on an individual's health or the moral rights of people to access information held by the state (for a useful summary, see McWhinnie, 2001). The discussion about the use of evidence reflected the growing preoccupation with evidence-based policy and practice elsewhere and two of our members, together with an overseas colleague (all social workers) produced a challenging paper which documented the different standards of evidence that were applied to policy development in social and emotional wellbeing against those used in medical science (Blyth, Crawshaw & Daniels, 2004).

Where appropriate, members identified themselves primarily by their role in Progar; when speaking or writing in a professional capacity through their employee positions, they sought to reference Progar where possible. The opportunity for open, internal debate within Progar was particularly important in helping individual members to develop their reflections and actions in a field where their direct work tended to take place in relative isolation.

## *Establishment of an Educational Arm, ACER*

When a body is solely concerned with campaigning, there can run the danger that it is not taken to have a reflective aspect to its work nor to draw on a credible body of evidence. Progar wished to counter this and decided that there was a strategic value in developing an educational arm which could provide educational seminars and literature. It therefore established ACER (Assisted Conception Education Resources Forum) in 2001 to fulfil this function and was immediately successful in obtaining a grant to run seminars for multi-disciplinary audiences drawn from within the assisted conception field but also from the wider social work, health, legal and child and family welfare communities in different parts of the UK throughout 2002-3. The presenters were primarily from a social work background (speaking on adoption, surrogacy and identity development) together with a lawyer and, in keeping with social work principles, the parent of donor conceived children drawing on her personal experience.

## *Development of Campaigning Literature*

The early part of BASW's work had seen the production of a booklet called 'Truth and the Child' (Bruce, Mitchell & Priestley, 1988) which was designed to influence the debate. Progar decided that the time had come to update that publication and a fuller book (with short individual pieces that were accessible both to the general reader and to the media) was produced, edited by three Progar members and published by BASW (Blyth, Crawshaw & Speirs, 1998). It included a mixture of personal and professional accounts and aimed to reflect the diversity of arguments for openness including social work, medical, genetic, sociological, psychological and legal.

Progar next turned its attention to its promotional literature. An earlier leaflet describing its work and principles was updated, taking care to achieve a more professional image. A new strap line 'Working to improve the law and services associated with assisted conception treatments' was agreed. The process proved a useful catalyst for discussion and debate and the reaffirming of its 2 key campaigning targets of:

- the right of people with fertility difficulties to informed choice and quality of care, including counselling, and
- the right of people to have access to identifying information about their genetic origins

In 2003, Progar again built on its earlier literature to produce a series of Briefing Papers, designed to highlight its broad membership and again with a professional image to enhance their readability and credibility. They included:

1. Overview Paper
2. Anonymous and Secret Donation: The legal position
3. The recruitment of identifiable sperm donors: Messages from overseas
4. Some useful psychological perspectives for thinking about donor conception in families

5. Medical indications for providing access to identifying information about gamete donors

The papers were variously authored by Progar members or invited authors and subject to an internal Progar editorial process. They were distributed to the media and influential figures from their introduction onwards and were then distributed through BASW to all members of the House of Commons and House of Lords during crucial Parliamentary processes in 2003/4 (see below).

### Building a Relationship with the HFEA

During the 1990s, Progar's links and dialogue with the HFEA developed. This included giving evidence to a number of public consultations run by the HFEA such those on the payment of donors and sex selection, taking the decision to invite a member of the HFEA executive to attend their meetings as observer, as already indicated, and holding regular meetings with them (see below). Despite earlier opposition to the lifting of anonymity, the HFEA finally came down in favour of the lifting of anonymity in 2002 when responding to the DH's consultation (see below) and we believe that this was in some measure due to Progar's activities.

Progar members made (and continue to make) increasingly diverse contributions to the work of the Authority:

- Three members of Progar became members of the HFEA's teams of clinic inspectors (though they were appointed independently of their role in Progar). This experience brought a vital perspective to Progar's work, especially in relation to clinics' attitudes towards psycho-social matters and the provision of counselling.
- In the late 1990s a liaison group was set up between the HFEA, the British Infertility Counselling Association (BICA) and Progar. All sides have valued these meetings which take place on a quarterly basis.
- One member of Progar was appointed as a member of the HFEA in 2003 (though again not as a Progar representative).

### ADDRESSING THE HFEA ANNUAL CONFERENCE– WHY ANONYMITY?

In December 2001, there had come a major breakthrough when EW was invited as Chair of Progar to give a keynote address to the HFEA's annual conference. She chose the title for her paper of 'Why Anonymity?' seeking to turn on its head the presumption that anonymity–staying with the status quo–was a safe and justifiable option. Progar's work had come a long way from the time when the issues on which we were campaigning were received in the field of assisted conception with a good deal of scorn and ridicule; when references to adoption were roundly refuted as having no transferable messages of value; and when social work was scapegoated as irrelevant and lacking in credibility.

## Some Key Themes of the 'Why Anonymity Paper'

### Views of Donor Conceived People

The presentation started with bringing the voices of those directly affected into the room in order to present the lifelong social and emotional nature of the outcomes to donor assisted conception treatment. David Gollancz (a member of Progar) on learning at age 12 that he had been conceived using donor sperm said: 'Being told that I had been conceived using a stranger's sperm was like being hit by a train. It didn't hurt. I wasn't angry or grief stricken or excited. I felt annihilated' (Gollancz, 2001:167).

Christine Whipp, a donor conceived woman who learned of her origins at age 41 said in the book co-edited by 3 Progar members: 'I have been cheated out of a proper family and created as a second class citizen, illegitimate and with no right to any information about my genealogical roots or family or medical history' (Whipp, 1998:64).

### The Impact of Secrecy

In 1988, Haimes wrote about the difficulties of accessing information about the impact of secrecy following donor conception when she said: 'However, the empirical evidence is weak so far, if only because we do not have access to the data. In that way secrecy carries within itself its own triumph since it prevents access to data through which it might be challenged' (p. 7). However, while not yet extensive, there is mounting evidence of its potential to damage, including in an important research study conducted by Turner and Coyle where Jessica's words illustrate the distress experienced on learning of genetic origins through accidental disclosure:

I was shocked and unforgiving. I now have a total distrust for my mother, and have realised that it is very hard for me to totally trust someone else. (Turner and Coyle 2000: 2045)

Sometimes the secret about a person's conception emerges in crisis and in an unplanned and damaging manner. There is increasing anecdotal evidence of problems occurring, for example, if there is a dispute between, or relationship break up of, the social parents, or if parents are asked in medical encounters for a family history particularly if the child develops an inherited disorder.

*Who Else Knows?*

There are worrying data about information being withheld from donor conceived children even though family and friends have been told. Golombok and Murray's study in 1999 interviewed, among others, 45 families with a child conceived through donor insemination. None had told their children about their origins although 51% had told the maternal grandparents, 20% had told paternal grandparents and 30% had told friends, giving rise to the potential for accidental or unplanned disclosure by a third party, distress and misunderstandings.

*Whose Needs?*

There is still a stigma attached to infertility and this drives many people to try to shelter behind secrecy. Hunter, Salter-Ling and Glover in their study of the experience of parents telling their children about their origins pointed out that '. . . secrecy serves to protect donors, doctors and parents needs rather than the needs of the child and may also be a response to the stigma of male infertility' (2000:157).

*Legal Issues*

There are three significant pieces of legislation and conventions that affect the debate in the UK:

- 1989 UN Convention on the Rights of the Child
- 1950 European Convention for the Protection of Human Rights and Fundamental Freedoms
- The Human Rights Act 1998 (UK)

Douglas, Lavery and Plumtree (1998) argued 'The international law, though ambiguous, case law and the experience of the working of the adoption legislation all point towards a growing acceptance that discovery of one's genetic identity is something which should be facilitated, rather than obstructed, by the law, It is likely that, in the next millennium, this acceptance will be extended to the position of children born after gamete donation. Until that occurs, the law remains complicated, inconsistent and unfair' (p. 13).

Challenges were outlined that were starting to be mounted in the courts (for example Joanna Rose, EM V The Secretary of State for Health and the Human Fertilisation and Embryology Authority) which, though still small in number, have impacted significantly on public opinion and increased pressure on the Government to lift anonymity. It was suggested that, pragmatically, changes would be likely to be forced through eventually with the Human Rights Act used increasingly to mount such challenges.

*Parallels with Adoption*

While the issues faced by people who have been adopted are not identical to those of donor conceived people there are sufficient similarities for lessons to be learned.

Evidence from adoption, together with the limited but growing research and anecdotal evidence in the field of donor conception, increasingly suggests that people denied knowledge of the identity and/or detailed knowledge of their genetic parents can feel cheated, deprived and incomplete. In adoption, there is growing evidence that those adopted in infancy may be looking for a completion of their identity when seeking out birth relatives rather than seeking substitute parental relationships. Even those who count themselves to be emotionally secure with close loving relationship with adoptive parents are showing a tendency to seek information and/or contact (Howe and Feast, 2000)– and those relationships appear to remain intact even when contact with birth parents is re-established. In an article looking to identify any potential parallels between the expressed needs of donor conceived people and adopted people, Crawshaw (2002) summarised the position for adopted people thus: 'Adopted people viewed their birth parents as people whom they wanted to know about, rather than simply as genetic vehicles' (p. 8) and concluded that the comparison with published accounts of the experiences of donor conceived people suggested important overlaps.

### Messages from Donor Conceived People

The presentation returned to the words of those most keenly affected: donor conceived people.

Rachel, who took part in the Turner and Coyle study, said: 'I needed to know whose face I was looking at in the mirror–I needed to know who I was and how I came to be–it was a very primal and unrelenting force which propelled the search and it was inescapable and undeniable (Turner & Coyle, 2000:2046).

Priscilla from the Donor Conception Support Group of Australia said: 'I'm not looking for a father figure; I already have one. The man who raised me is my Dad as far as I'm concerned but it would be nice to know who gave me the gift of life. Until I find him a part of me is missing' (Donor Conception Support Group of Australia newsletter, 2000).

### Key Questions

EW concluded by posing the following key questions:

- Are secrets damaging and dangerous?
- Is it right to deceive people?
- Do you teach your children to be honest? How do you feel when you catch them out in a lie?
- Is it right to discriminate in law against donor offspring?
- Is it right to deny donor conceived people access to information held about them by the state?
- Where does the balance lie of the moral and civil rights of all parties concerned?

## THE ROLE OF THE BRITISH ASSOCIATION OF SOCIAL WORKERS

Throughout the whole of this time, Progar remained under the sponsoring umbrella of BASW and retained its full support. Crucially, BASW recognised the fact that Progar had come to have some members who were neither social workers nor BASW members and recognised that it remained appropriate to remain the parent organisation and provide support.

## The Significance of Underpinning Principles

The International Federation of Social Workers and the International Association of Schools of Social Work define social work as follows:

> The social work profession promotes social change, problem solving in human relationships and the empowerment and liberation of people to enhance well-being. Utilising theories of human behaviour and social systems, social work intervenes at the points where people interact with their environments. Principles of human rights and social justice are fundamental to social work. (2001)

The BASW Code of Ethics (2002) is committed to five basic values of human dignity and worth, social justice, service to humanity, integrity and competence. It further argues that every human being has intrinsic value and that all persons have a right to well-being, to self-fulfilment and to as much control over their own lives as is consistent with the rights of others. Alongside respecting basic human rights, the BASW Code sets out social workers' duty to:

> Safeguard and promote service users dignity, individuality, rights, responsibilities and identity (3.1.2.c)

and to:

> Bring to the attention of those in power and the general public, and where appropriate challenge ways in which the policies or activities of government, organisations or society create or contribute to structural disadvantage, hardship and suffering, or militate against their relief (3.2.2.a) Seek to change social structures which perpetuate inequalities and injustices, and whenever possible work to eliminate all violations of human rights (3.2.2.c) and Challenge the abuse of power for suppression and for excluding people from decisions which affect them. (3.2.2.f)

In keeping with this, Progar's work has been built around the principle that it is a fundamental moral and human right that people should not be denied information about their genetic origins, where it is known. As donor conceived people have not asked to be conceived and, since they cannot advocate for themselves at the point of conception or their entry into society as infants, we have argued that society must ensure the primacy of their needs.

However, Progar also believes that the rights and needs of infertile people and donors are important and that it is unhelpful, unconstructive and against core social work values to collude with debates that seek to polarise the rights of those in intimate relationships with each other and construct them as being 'good' and 'bad,' 'deserving' and 'undeserving.' By increasingly seeking to locate its arguments within a child welfare, family and social context, Progar sought to challenge the polarising tendency. In keeping with the need to attend to psycho-social needs as experienced in the here and now while actively engaging in the political debate, Progar has also consistently advocated the need for counselling and support services provided by qualified professionals to be made available to all parties throughout their lifetime.

## *WINNING HEARTS AND MINDS*

The lifting of or retaining the anonymity of gamete donors, and indeed the whole subject of infertility, is an emotive subject which generates strongly held views. Historically, some of the medical community have voiced the most strongly held views against the lifting of anonymity. Some of these views are driven by economic and professional self-interest where the fear is held that donor supplies would reduce with the lifting of anonymity. Some are no doubt related to individuals' personal involvement through their own past donations while others firmly feel that maintaining secrecy is beneficial to family life and parent-child relationships.

Scare stories, typically in the tabloid press, have focussed on the potential for the reduction of sperm donor numbers though rarely on egg donor supply–an intriguing gendered dimension. International evidence suggests that sperm donor numbers do indeed reduce initially but then gradually increase again with an older, more mature donor coming forward–though this remains a hotly contested area. Sometimes, the focus of the tabloid press has been on the spectre of donor conceived people turning up on the donor's doorstep demanding money or some form of legal rights. The supply/demand arguments rarely engage in debating the lifelong moral or psycho-social aspects of the families affected (either those containing a donor conceived offspring or those of the donor) but hoist their colours firmly to the consumerist arguments of the couple seeking donor conception treatment and the clinic who wishes to supply them.

However, there has been a gradual but noticeable shift in attitudes. Changing attitudes to openness and children's rights within wider society and the awareness of the damage caused by secrets and accidental disclosure are now written and spoken about more openly and another, more reflective form of media coverage through television and the quality newspapers has come to the fore. There has been an accompanying gradual shift away from a technical or medicalised approach to infertility to one where infertility is seen more in terms of the lifetime needs and rights of the families to be formed or affected. There has been an increasing recognition of the appropriateness of drawing an analogy with adoption, in part due to the increasing recognition of the validity of professional practice and research experience in social work.

When giving the paper at the HFEA conference in 2001, EW anticipated, based on previous experience, that she would encounter much more opposition than she did. Instead, the discussion focussed on when and how to lift anonymity rather than whether or not to. Times were changing.

## THE SITUATION TODAY

Section 31 of the HFE Act required that Regulations be laid before Parliament in preparation for the first donor conceived people having the right to consult the Register of Information in 2008. After several false starts, the DH finally launched a consultation exercise in December 2001 to determine how non-identifying information should be handled and whether and how anonymity should be lifted. If it was to be lifted prospectively (and this was what Progar campaigned for), it would only require secondary legislation. The most crucial part yet of Progar's long campaigning activity was about to commence.

Progar undertook its campaign in a variety of ways including running a conference with an invited audience in May 2002 generously funded by the internationally recognised Nuffield Foundation. Invitations were drawn up on the basis of influencing a wide range of professional and political opinion. The conference explored the importance of lifting anonymity from the point of view of donor conceived people and social parents and from a medical, genetic, legal and social work perspective. Baroness Warnock, with whom Progar had developed a dialogue in recent years and who had joined its campaign to lobby for change, gave the keynote address which ensured high national media coverage. She used this platform to announce publicly that she had changed her mind about donor anonymity and why. She stated her belief that withholding identifying information represented the denial of a fundamental moral right for every donor conceived person and that she and the Warnock Committee had not foreseen that their acceptance of donor anonymity would have led to parents withholding vital information about the circumstances of their child's conception from them. Her announcement was an extremely important contribution to the consultation process and attracted, as anticipated, a great deal of media attention.

Progar subsequently gained a meeting with the then Public Health Minister, Hazel Blears.

In January 2003, the Government announced at the HFEA Annual Conference that they accepted in principle the need for openness and for the paramountcy of the welfare of the children affected but, frustratingly, also said that they needed more time to arrive at a final decision about the lifting of anonymity and set up an additional six month research period. In the same speech, the Minister announced the establishment of the piloting of a UK voluntary information exchange and contact register for people conceived prior to August 1991. The work was awarded to After Adoption Yorkshire, and UK DonorLink (www.ukdonorlink.org.uk) was established and launched in April 2004, with MC (a Progar member) acting as Adviser and Chair of the Advisory Group in her professional capacity.

Individual Progar members contributed extensively to the DH's work during the period that was set aside for additional research as did Progar as a group. A year later, with a change of Public Health Minister to Melanie Johnson and a meeting between her and Progar, came the announcement that Progar had been waiting for. On 21st January 2004, Melanie Johnson announced that the Government would be putting in place a process that would change the legislation and come into force in April 2005, lifting anonymity prospectively. From that date, donors were to donate in the knowledge that their identity would be open and known from the age of majority of any person whose conception resulted from their donation. Work continued following the announcement including:

- Drafting the Regulations and taking them through Parliament
- Determining how to handle the interim period

- Determining how to allow people who had already donated to alter their consent to allow for openness
- Deciding how to promote openness and a change in culture in treatment centres and amongst the public
- Continuing to address the rights and needs of the families affected

The Government has undertaken publicity initiatives and worked with organisations such as the National Gamete Donation Trust, British Fertility Society, UK DonorLink and, of course, Progar to encourage new and existing donors to come forward and to embed the new culture of openness into services.

## CURRENT AND FUTURE CHALLENGES

The challenges in this ethically and socially complex field of work continue. There are a myriad of aspects of donor conception and assisted conception that need to be addressed. The lifetime implications continue to unfold. The scandalous lack of services to either prospective or existing parents to enable them to be supported in telling their children of their conception and coping with the associated parenting demands together with the lack of support services for existing donor conceived people (children and adults) and donors continue to make those affected vulnerable. The needs of donor conceived people who still have no rights to access their records and the needs of those who find out in accidental or unplanned ways at any stage in their lives continue to be of concern. And the ongoing tension between, on the one hand, the commercialisation and commodification of family building and, on the other, the desire to engage in emotionally and socially healthy family building ensures that Progar's role will continue to be needed.

## CONCLUSION

Social work traditionally concerns itself with vulnerable groups and actively seeks to promote the need to attend to, and challenge, the social context within which vulnerability is formed and maintained. Engaging with issues around assisted conception stems from a long tradition within medical social work in particular of seeing those receiving medical attention as people and social beings first and foremost and thus resisting the medicalisation of social experience. Many of the families formed through donor conception treatment enjoy socio-economic privilege as economically deprived groups (who typically are *over*-represented among users of social work services) often find themselves unable to access these treatments. The ability of Progar and the social workers within it to see vulnerability without its traditional socioeconomic mantle has proved vital to the campaign in which it has engaged.

There are many different stakeholders in this debate. Their political and theoretical orientations have contributed to the polarisation of the arguments. Social work has shown itself here, as elsewhere in its history, to have the potential to bridge those divides and maintain core attention to the lived experience in its social and historical context. Crucially, it sees beyond individualised explanations which reduce and narrow understanding in order to resist the medicalisation or pathologising of experience.

In the current UK social work context, the shift towards the care management social policy agenda in recent years has placed enormous pressure on the profession to adopt a more bureaucratic, consumerist approach to its task. In consequence, medical social work has been pushed towards an undue emphasis on discharge planning out of a predominantly welfare context with people who can afford to buy their own care being increasingly excluded from access to social work services. The need to hold firm on social work principles and values is perhaps more crucial than ever. Progar's campaign illustrates the importance of seeing the individual/family/social group and their need in context (whether that be predominantly socio-economic or not) and to attend to them within that perspective *at the same time* as engaging with the policy makers and opinion formers to influence that wider social context.

It is difficult to say how far the other players recognise the social work contribution to the campaign to lift anonymity and it is not the focus of this paper to evaluate its relative influence. However, it is interesting and validating that the Vice Chair of the HFEA recently wrote: 'Although the HFEA supported this change, it was primarily urged by the social work profession in the light of their experience. . . .' (Baldwin, 2005:84).

## NOTE ON THE UK LEGISLATIVE PROCESS

When considering legislation a topic is proposed by the Government of the day and discussed in Parliament. The government then produces a Green Paper which may be handled in a variety of ways but is generally discussed in Parliamentary Committees. There may be a preceding or succeeding public consultation. A White Paper is then produced and handled in a similar way. The legislation is then drafted and comes before Parliament as a Bill. It will go before the House of Commons and the House of Lords and will often go back and forth between the two Houses, debating and agreeing or rejecting amendments. Some of the earlier stages may be foreshortened. The final legislation known as the Act becomes law after it has received Royal Assent, which is a formality.

Most Acts of Parliament have subsequent regulations and guidance, some of which require Parliamentary consideration.

## REFERENCES

Baldwin T (2005) 'Ethical issues in a changing world' *Human Fertility* Vol 8 No 2 June 2005, 83-89.

Blyth E, Crawshaw M & Speirs J (eds) (1998) *Truth and the Child–Information Exchange in Donor Assisted Conception* Venture Press, Birmingham

Blyth ED, Crawshaw MA & Daniels K (2004) Policy formation in gamete donation and egg sharing in the UK–A critical appraisal *Social Science and Medicine* 59(2004) 2617-2626

Blyth E & Hunt J (1998) 'Sharing genetic origins information in donor assisted conception: Views from licensed centres on HFEA donor information form (91) 4' *Human Reproduction* Vol 13 no 11 pp 3274-3277

Bruce N, Mitchell A & Priestley K (1988) *Truth and the Child* Edinburgh, Family Care

Crawshaw M A (2002) 'Lessons from a recent adoption study to identify some of the service needs of, and issues for, donor offspring wanting to know about their donors' in *Human Fertility* Vol 5 No 1 Feb 2002, 6-12

Donor Conception Support Group of Australia (1997) *Let the Offspring Speak–Discussions on Donor Conception* The Donor Conception Support Group of Australia, PO Box 53, Georges Hall, New South Wales 2198, Australia

Donor Conception Support Group of Australia Newsletter (2000) The Donor Conception Support Group of Australia, PO Box 53, Georges Hall, New South Wales 2198, Australia

Douglas G, Lavery R & Plumtree A (1998) 'Truth and the Child: The legal perspective' in *Blyth E, Crawshaw M and Speirs J (1998) op cit*

Gollancz D (2001) 'Donor insemination: A question of rights' *Human Fertility* (2001) 4 164-167

Golombok S & Murray (1999) 'Social versus biological parenting: Family functioning and the socioemotional development of children conceived by egg or sperm donation' in *Journal of Child Psychology and Psychiatry* Vol 40 No 4 pp 519-527

Haimes E (1998) 'Truth and the child: A sociological perspective' in *Blyth E, Crawshaw M and Speirs J (1998) op cit*

Howe D & Feast J (2000) *Adoption, Search & Reunion–The Long Term Experience of Adopted Adults* The Children's Society, London

Hunter M, Salter-Ling N & Glover L (2000) 'Donor insemination: Telling children about their origins' *Child Psychology & Psychiatry Review* Volume 5 No 4 pp. 157-156

McWhinnie A (2001) 'Should offspring from donated gametes continue to be denied knowledge of their origins and antecedents?' *Human Reproduction* Vol 16 No 5 pp 807-817

Turner A & Coyle A (2000) 'What does it mean to be a donor offspring? The identity experiences of adults conceived by donor insemination and the implications for counselling and therapy' *Human Reproduction* Vol 15 No 9 2041-2051

Warnock M (1984) *A Question of Life: The Warnock Report on Human Fertilisation and Embryology* Oxford, Basil Blackwell

Whipp C (1998) 'The legacy of deceit: A donor offspring's perspective on secrecy in assisted conception' *in Blyth E, Crawshaw M and Speirs J (1998) op cit*

# Caregiving Stressors and Psychological Distress Among Veteran Resident and Immigrant Family Caregivers in Israel

Varda Soskolne, PhD
Sara Halevy-Levin, MSW
Ann Cohen, BSW
Gideon Friedman, MD

**SUMMARY.** The study compared caregiving stressors and psychological distress between Israeli veteran resident and immigrant family caregivers. It examined whether psychosocial variables (appraisal of caregiving, mastery, social support and coping) mediate the differences

Varda Soskolne is affiliated with the School of Social Work, Bar-Ilan University, Ramat-Gan, Israel and the School of Public Health, Hadassah-Hebrew University Medical Center, Jerusalem, Israel. Sara Halevy-Levin is affiliated with the Department of Social Work Services, and the Geriatric Unit, Department of Medicine, Hadassah-Hebrew University Medical Center, Jerusalem, Israel. Ann Cohen is affiliated with the Department of Social Work Services, Hadassah-Hebrew University Medical Center, Jerusalem, Israel. Gideon Friedman is affiliated with the Geriatric Unit, Department of Medicine, Hadassah-Hebrew University Medical Center, Jerusalem, Israel.

Address correspondence to: Varda Soskolne, PhD, School of Social Work, Bar-Ilan University, Ramat-Gan 52900 Israel (E-mail: varda@vms.huji.ac.il).

The authors thank the staff of the home-care units of Maccabi, Meuhedet, Leumit and Clalit Health Services, and of the Geriatric Unit, Hospice Home Care Unit and the Retired Personnel Services of Hadassah University Hospitals for their assistance.

The study was funded by the Chief Scientist Office, Israel Ministry of Health (# 4745).

[Haworth co-indexing entry note]: "Caregiving Stressors and Psychological Distress Among Veteran Resident and Immigrant Family Caregivers in Israel." Soskolne et al. Co-published simultaneously in *Social Work in Health Care* (The Haworth Press, Inc.) Vol. 43, No. 2/3, 2006, pp. 73-93; and: *International Social Health Care Policy, Programs, and Studies* (ed: Gary Rosenberg, and Andrew Weissman) The Haworth Press, Inc., 2006, pp. 73-93. Single or multiple copies of this article are available for a fee from The Haworth Document Delivery Service [1-800-HAWORTH, 9:00 a.m. - 5:00 p.m. (EST). E-mail address: docdelivery@haworthpress.com].

Available online at http://swhc.haworthpress.com
© 2006 by The Haworth Press, Inc. All rights reserved.
doi:10.1300/J010v43n02_06

in psychological distress between these two groups. A total of 213 veteran resident and 206 immigrant (from the former Soviet Union) caregivers of chronically ill elderly were recruited from health services. The comparisons between the two groups were examined separately for spouse and adult child caregivers. The immigrant spouse and adult child caregivers reported significantly higher levels of caregiving stressors than veteran resident caregivers, but psychological distress was significantly higher only among the immigrant adult child caregivers. In multivariate analyses, the difference in psychological distress disappeared when caregiving stressors and mediating psychosocial variables were included in the regression models. Different caregiving stressors and psychosocial variables were associated with psychological distress among the spouses and among the adult child caregivers. The findings suggest that the caregiving stressors and psychosocial variables explain differences in psychological health outcomes between veteran resident and immigrant caregivers. Social work interventions should address these factors among caregivers, take into account the relationship to the care recipient, be culturally adapted to the immigrant caregivers, and target immigrant adult child caregivers in particular. *[Article copies available for a fee from The Haworth Document Delivery Service: 1-800-HAWORTH. E-mail address: <docdelivery@haworthpress.com> Website: <http://www.HaworthPress. com> © 2006 by The Haworth Press, Inc. All rights reserved.]*

**KEYWORDS.** Family caregiving, psychological distress, immigrants, Israel

## INTRODUCTION

In the rapidly growing literature on family caregiving, research on ethnic and cultural differences is relatively limited (Dilworth-Anderson, Williams, & Gibson, 2002). The majority of the studies examine racial differences between White and Black caregivers (Farran, Miller, Kaufman, & Davis, 1997; Haley, Roth, Coleton, Ford, West, Collins, & Isobe, 1996; Lawton, Rajagopal, Brody, & Kleban, 1992; Miller, Campbell, Farran, Kaufman, & Davis, 1995; White, Townsend, & Stephens Parris, 2000), while fewer include other ethnic groups, such as Latino, Asian American or non-American (Aranda & Knight, 1997; Patterson, Semple, Shaw, Yu, He, Zhang et al., 1998: Youn, Knight,

Jeong, & Benton, 1999). A recent review stressed the need to differentiate the diversity within the White populations in order to identify distinct cultural and ethnic identities that may influence a family's approach to caregiving for its dependent elder members (Dilworth-Anderson et al., 2002). In Israel, a multi ethnic society, with recent waves of mass immigration from different cultural backgrounds, little is known about the cultural differences in family caregiving context and outcomes in terms of physical and psychological health. Given the increased aging of the Israeli population and the high proportion of the chronically ill elderly among recent immigrants from the former Soviet Union (FSU) (Brodsky, 1998), the need for assistance in personal care is expected to grow, and with it–the burden on family members who provide the majority of care at home. Understanding these cultural differences is, therefore, particularly important. The current study, based on the transactional theoretical model of stress and coping (Lazarus & Folkman, 1984), and its application to caregiving stress (Pearlin, Mullan, Semple, & Skaff, 1990), examined differences in caregiving stressors and health outcomes between two culturally distinct groups– immigrants from the FSU and established veteran Israelis.[1]

### *Caregiving Stressors, Mediators, and Psychological Distress*

According to the stress and coping model (Lazarus & Folkman, 1984), the association of stressors with health outcomes is mediated by cognitive appraisal of the stressors and subsequent coping processes. Antecedent person and social resources are directly associated with health outcomes and often moderate the association of stressors with health (Lazarus & Folkman, 1984; Thoits, 1995). Family caregiving is, generally, a prolonged stressful situation in which caregivers' stressors arise from the wide range of care activities provided to disabled or demented patients at home (Tennstedt, 1999). Caregiving stressors, such as the degree of disability of the care recipient and caregiving tasks, have been associated with elevated levels of distress and depressive affect (Tennstedt, 1999; Yates, Tennstedt, & Chang, 1999). Direct and mediating or moderating effects of personal and social resources, caregiving appraisal and coping on the association between caregiving stress and psychological health have been identified (Bookwala & Schulz, 1998; Haley et al., 1996; Li, Seltzer, & Greenberg, 1997; Patterson et al., 1998; Tennstedt, 1999). Some studies have shown that the mediating role of appraisal is better understood when it is differentiated between negative appraisal of caregiving–that correlated with higher depression scores (Yates et al., 1999), and positive appraisal that correlated with lower distress (Haley et al., 1996; Noonan & Tennstedt, 1997). Greater use of coping strategies for management of distress (emotion-focused) was associated with elevated emotional distress or depression (Li et al., 1997), while management of the situation (problem-focused coping) was associated with lower distress (Folkman, 1997). Among caregivers, since the care recipient status is often irreversible, coping efforts aim not only to make the situation more manageable but also to manage the meaning of caregiving (Pearlin et al., 1990), constantly reappraising the situation (Folkman, 1997).

Different cultural backgrounds may shape all the factors in the model and precipitate diverse stress outcome since the cognitive appraisal of the stressor is determined not only by its characteristics but also by the individual's norms, beliefs and psychological resources (Lazarus & Folkman, 1984). Cultural norms thus influence the mediating variables–caregiving appraisal, the use of support systems and coping behaviors, indirectly having an impact on health outcomes (Haley et al., 1996; Patterson et al., 1998; Young & Kahana, 1995): a sociocultural stress and coping process (Aranda & Knight, 1997). Yet, there are still considerable inconsistencies (Dilworth-Anderson et al., 2002).

Relation to care recipient (e.g., spouse or child) is a significant factor in the caregiving stress model. It was found to be an important determinant of overload appraisal (Yates et al., 1999), social support (Li et al., 1997) and psychological outcomes, with spouses generally showing greater psychological distress than adult child caregivers (Pot, Deeg, van Dyck, & Jonker, 1998; Tennstedt, 1999).

### Caregiving in Israel Among Veteran Residents and Immigrants

In Israel, most of the disabled patients are eligible for formal home-care services under the Community Long-term Care Law. Yet, these services are not sufficient to meet all the needs. Due to the strong family ties characteristic of Israeli society (Walter-Ginzburg et al., 2001), elderly in need of assistance with daily living activities at home often benefit from informal care. Family members provide most (80%) of the assistance but feel the burden to be too high (Brodsky, 1998). Positive attitudes, such as filial responsibility (Litwin, 1994), and lower perceived harmful effects (Kulik, 2001) contribute to higher rates of family caregiving. So far, data on caregiving stressors and their association with health outcomes, particularly in diverse cultural context, are scarce.

A recent wave of immigration from the FSU to Israel since 1989 added close to 1 million people to the existing population. These Jewish immigrants are marked by a very distinct cultural background, and by the long-standing experience of an authoritative, closed society, features that distinguish them from the veteran Israeli population and mark them as a group (Ben-Rafael, Olshtain, & Geijst, 1997, p. 364). In addition, the immigrants are characterized by a higher proportion of elderly people (Brodsky, 1998), chronic disease (Nirel, Rosen, Gross, Berg, & Youval, 1996), and disabilities (Strosberg & Naon, 1997), suggesting a higher need for informal caregiving. While co-residence with the elderly was common in the FSU (Mirsky, 1998), and a strong moral and cultural norm motivated many to support and care for the sick or disabled elderly within the family (Remennick, 1999), even more families share households following immigration due to economic constraints (Strosberg & Naon, 1997). The sick or disabled elderly often became more dependent on younger family members, particularly daughters and daughters-in-law, themselves struggling with adjustment difficulties (Remennick, 2001). These cultural attitudes towards caregiving for the elderly, combined with economic and social difficulties not prevalent among veteran Israeli caregivers, may contribute to greater caregiving stressors, and to distinct stress and coping processes and health outcomes among the immigrants.

Hence, the aim of this study was to compare caregiving stress and health outcomes between two cultural groups (defined by immigration status) of family caregivers to chronically ill elderly. Specifically, it aimed (1) To compare the caregiving stressors, personal and social resources, caregiving appraisal, and coping and psychological distress outcomes between the caregiver groups (veteran residents and immigrants); and (2) To examine the contribution of caregiving stressors and psychosocial mediating variables (negative and positive appraisal of caregiving, mastery, social support and coping) to differences in psychological distress between the two groups. Based on previous empirical evidence of differences in caregiving stressors and outcomes between spouses and adult children (Li et al., 1997; Tennstedt, 1999), these comparisons were examined separately for each relationship type.

## METHODS

### Design and Procedures

The participants for this cross-sectional comparative study were recruited during the year 2001 from the home-care units of the four

Health Maintenance Organizations in Jerusalem, and from three ambulatory units of the Hadassah Hospitals (the Geriatric Unit, Hospice Home Care Unit and the Retired Personnel Services). *Inclusion criteria*: (a) Care recipient–aged 55 years or older, in need of assistance with two or more activities of daily living (ADL), and/or instrumental ADL (IADL), or in need of constant supervision. (b) Primary family caregivers who provide care on a regular basis for at least 5 weekly hours and for two months or more. (c) First-kin family caregivers (spouses, children, children-in-law), 25 years of age or older, independent in ADL and IADL, veteran Israeli residents (Israeli-born or residents in Israel for 20 years or more) or immigrants from the FSU who arrived since 1990.

Having received approval of Human Subjects Committees, names of caregivers were selected from lists of eligible patients being cared for by each service. The number of family members involved in caregiving at each service could be established only after an initial contact. In two services (the Hospice Home Care and the Hadassah Retired Personnel Unit) all the eligible caregivers were included. In the other services, consecutive samples of Israeli or immigrant caregivers were selected to reach about 15-30% of the potential populations. Having signed an informed consent form, the participants were interviewed at home in Hebrew or Russian by trained interviewers. A total of 588 eligible family members were approached of whom 419 (71%) were interviewed, 213 (66%) veteran and 206 (79%) immigrant caregivers. The main reasons for non-response were refusal (19%) and lack of time (9%). The non-participants differed from the participants in their relationship to care recipient but not in age or gender. The proportion of spouses among the non-participants (56%) was higher than among the participants (41.5%).

### *Measures*

#### *Demographics*

*Caregiver demographics* included the relationship to care recipient, age, gender, marital status (for non-spouse caregivers), education, family income, country of birth, employment, and years in Israel. *Care recipient demographics* included age and gender.

#### *Caregiving Stressors*

*(a) Care recipient status* was measured by several well-established scales. Higher scores represent greater impairment. *Functional status*

was measured by the 5-item Activities of Daily Living (ADL) scale and a 5-item Instrumental Activities of Daily Living (IADL) scale (Fillenbaum, 1985). The mean ADL score ranges between 0 to 2.2 and mean IADL score ranges between 0 to 1, with Cronbach's alpha were 0.83 and 0.76 for ADL and IADL, respectively, and were similar in both groups. *Cognitive impairment* was measured by an 8-item scale (Pearlin et al., 1990). Cronbach's alpha was 0.94 and was similar in both groups. *Problem behavior* was measured by responses to the frequency of five behaviors (wandering, yelling or cursing, hitting, acting inappropriately, or accusing others of stealing) adapted from Yates et al. (1999). Each item ranges from 0 'never' to 4 'very often' but due to the skewness of the distribution the summative scale was not used and it was further dichotomized to 0 'none' and 1 'any problem behavior.'

*(b) Caregiving tasks* were constructed specifically for the study as the mean value of the frequency of assistance in each of the ADL and IADL items, ranging from 1 'not at all' to 4 'all the time.' Cronbach's alphas were 0.76 and 0.78 for help with ADL and IADL, respectively, and were similar in both groups.

## Psychosocial Resources and Mediators

*Personal and social resources*: (a) Mastery–a 7-item scale that measures the sense of control over issues in a person's life (Pearlin & Schooler, 1978). Each item ranges from '1' to '4' (high mastery). Cronbach's alpha was 0.71 and similar in both groups. (b) *Social resources* were measured by the Medical Outcome Study (MOS) Social Support Scale, a 19-item scale tapping emotional, instrumental, tangible or affective support (Sherbourne-Donald & Stewart, 1991). The total score was used for the current study with higher scores representing greater support. Cronbach's alpha was 0.96 and similar in both groups.

*Appraisal of caregiving*: Appraisal of negative aspects was measured by two scales (Pearlin et al., 1990). *Role overload*–a 4-item scale, which indicates how much an individual feels overwhelmed by the tasks of caregiving. Cronbach's alpha was 0.80 and was similar in both groups. *Role captivity*–a 3-item scale that indicates the perception of being captive in the caregiving role. Cronbach's alpha was 0.78 and similar in both groups. Higher scores on both scales represent more negative appraisal. The positive aspect of caregiving was measured by *caregiving self-esteem*, i.e., the extent to which caregiving imparts individual self-esteem, a 7-item subscale, (Nijboer, Triemstra Tempelaar, Sanderman & van den Bos, 1999). Higher scores represent more positive appraisal. One item lowered the Cronbach's alpha and after it was deleted Cronbach's alpha was moderate among the immigrant caregivers (0.68), but low among the veteran caregivers (0.46).

*Coping strategies*: The participants were asked to report their use of various coping strategies in relation to a particular event they identified as the most stressful event related to caregiving. Five sub-scales (i.e., planful problem solving, positive reappraisal, escape-avoidance, seeking social support, and distancing) of the shortened version of the Ways of Coping Questionnaire (Folkman, Lazarus, Pimley, & Novacek, 1987) were chosen based on their relevance to caregiving (Moskowitz-Tedlie, Folkman, Collette, & Vittinghoff, 1996). Higher scores represent greater use of the strategy. Cronbach's alphas for most of the sub-scales were low to medium level, ranging between 0.48 to 0.66.

### Psychological Distress

The 24-item Talbieh Brief Distress Scale–TBDI (Ritsner, Rabinowitz, & Slyuzberg, 1995) in its Hebrew and Russian versions was used. The items were originally drawn from the well-known Brief Symptom Inventory (BSI) and the Psychiatric Epidemiology Research Interview Demoralization Scale (Peri-D) and are highly correlated with both scales. The total Distress Index, ranging from 0-4 with higher scores representing greater distress, was used in the current study. Cronbach's alpha was 0.91 and was similar in both groups. This scale was preferred over others because of its frequent use in studies of immigrants from the FSU (e.g., Ritsner & Ponizovsky, 1999; 2003).

### Statistical Analysis

Each cultural group was stratified by relationship to care-receiver: spouses vs. adult children, including children-in-law (who comprised only 8% of the veteran and 17% of immigrant samples). Exclusion of children-in-law did not change the results and they were retained in the analysis. Additionally, examining the cultural background of the veteran resident caregivers revealed that 54% of these spouses and 66% of these adult children were of European (Ashkenazi) origin, the rest of Middle Eastern origin. Selection of a comparison group comprised only of veteran Soviet immigrants (> 20 years) from within the veteran Israeli caregivers was not feasible. Therefore, we opted to retain all the veteran caregivers rather than to choose only Ashkenazi veteran residents (who are not of the same cultural background as the immigrants), in order to have a better representation of the general veteran resident caregivers.

Bivariate analyses were conducted to compare the distributions of the study variables between the groups. For multivariate analysis, hierarchical linear regression models (Cohen & Cohen, 1983) were performed to test the association of distress with group affiliation when other factors are accounted for. In model 1, group affiliation was entered alone followed by demographic control variables and caregiving stressors (model 2). Psychosocial resources (mastery and social support), caregiving appraisal, and coping were added in the last stage (model 3). Significance level for inclusion into the next stage was set at $p < 0.10$ in order to decrease the number of variables. Modifying effects of the psychosocial resources were examined by interaction terms with group affiliation.

## RESULTS

### Description of the Population

In both types of relationship to care recipient, small or non-significant differences were found between the veteran and immigrant caregivers in age, gender, marital status, and employment status but they differed significantly in number of children, education, and family income (Table 1). The immigrant caregivers had significantly higher education but lower levels of family income. The majority of the immigrant caregivers (67%) had already been living in Israel for more than 8 years.

The care receiver's age did not differ between the spouse groups (mean age was 73 in both groups), but immigrant adult child caregivers were caring for older care recipients (mean age 84.3, S.D. 7.7) than the veteran caregivers (mean age 81.6, S.D. 8.6, $p < 0.05$).

### Caregiving Stressors, Resources, Appraisal, Coping and Psychological Distress

Table 2 presents the comparison between the groups for each measure.

#### Caregiving Stressors

*Care recipient status*: Few differences in the care recipient status were found between the two groups. Among spouse caregivers, ADL and the cognitive status of the care recipients were more deteriorated among veteran residents. Among the parents of adult child caregivers the cognitive status of the immigrant parents was more deteriorated.

*Caregiving tasks*: While all the caregivers provided greater assistance with IADL than with ADL, the immigrant caregivers provided significantly more of these tasks than the veteran Israeli caregivers (not reaching statistical significance in help with ADL among the spouses).

## Personal and Social Resources

The level of mastery was higher among the immigrant than among the veteran spouse caregivers but no difference was found among the adult child caregivers. In contrast, the levels of social support were significantly lower among the immigrant caregivers in both relationship types than among the veteran caregivers.

## Caregiving Appraisal

While both the spouse and the adult child immigrant caregivers reported significantly higher levels of role overload than the veteran caregivers, they felt less captive in the caregiver role (reaching statistical significance only among the spouses). Regarding positive appraisal, the immigrant spouses reported greater caregiving self-esteem than the veteran spouses but the *opposite* direction was found among the adult child caregivers.

TABLE 1. Background characteristics of the two groups, by caregiver relationship

| Caregiver characteristics | Spouse caregivers | | Adult child caregivers | |
|---|---|---|---|---|
| | Veteran (N = 108) | Immigrant (N = 66) | Veteran (N = 105) | Immigrant (N = 140) |
| Age (mean, SD) | 69.7 (10.9) | 71.0 (9.46) | 51.3 (9.68) | 54.0 (10.6)* |
| Gender: women | 75% | 61% | 83% | 84% |
| Marital status: married | -- | -- | 68% | 64% |
| Education: less than high school | 64% | 17% *** | 36% | 16% *** |
| Employment: yes | 16% | 11% | 62% | 67% |
| Family monthly income: less than IS4500[a] | 31% | 85% *** | 25% | 39% ** |

[a] IS = Israeli Shekels (Equivalent to $1100 at the time of the study)
* P < 0.05  ** P < 0.01  ***P < 0.001

## Coping

The immigrant caregivers used significantly more coping strategies than the veteran caregivers. This was expressed in planful problem solving, reappraisal strategies and in emotion-focused coping by escape-avoidance but not by distancing. Only among the adult children, the veteran caregivers sought more support for assistance with caregiving problems.

## Psychological Distress

Psychological distress was higher among the immigrant caregivers but it reached statistical significance only among the adult child caregivers.

### Multivariate Analyses

For brevity, only the final models (stage 3) of the regressions, when all the variables are included, are presented. No significant interaction terms of group with caregiving appraisal and psychosocial resources were found.

*(a) Spouse caregivers*: The non-significant association of cultural group with psychological distress ($\beta = 0.09$ in the first stage) remained at all stages of the analysis. The final model (Table 3) shows that when income was controlled, the presence of problem behaviors was the only caregiving stressor that was significantly associated with psychological distress. Additionally, spouses with lower levels of mastery, those who appraised caregiving as more negative (higher role captivity) and coped by seeking less support and by lower distancing had significantly higher psychological distress. These psychosocial variables contributed close to 22% of the total 33% explained variance in psychological distress.

*(b) Adult child caregivers*: The initial significant higher level of psychological distress among the immigrant caregivers (model 1, $\beta = 0.12$, $p < 0.05$) disappeared once all the other variables were included (Table 3). Psychological distress was significantly higher when the care recipient had behavior problems, when he/she was *less* disabled in ADL, yet when the caregiver provided more assistance with ADL, when mastery was lower, when negative caregiving appraisal (role overload and captivity) was higher, and when coping by escape-avoidance was greater

TABLE 2. Comparison of caregiving stressors, psychosocial resources, caregiving appraisal, coping and health outcomes between veteran and immigrant caregivers

| Variable[a] | Spouse caregivers | | Adult child caregivers | |
|---|---|---|---|---|
| | Veteran (N = 108) | Immigrant (N = 66) | Veteran (N = 105) | Immigrant (N = 140) |
| Caregiving stressors | Mean (SD) | Mean (SD) | Mean (SD) | Mean (SD) |
| a. Care recipient status | | | | |
| ADL | 1.21 (0.67) | 0.93 (0.60)** | 1.14 (0.63) | 1.01 (0.62) |
| IADL | 0.96 (0.13) | 0.97 (0.09) | 0.95 (0.15) | 0.95 (0.18) |
| Problem behavior (any) | 35% | 42% | 45% | 55% |
| Cognitive status | 1.31 (1.37) | 0.84 (1.14)* | 1.05 (1.11) | 1.36 (1.25)* |
| b. Caregiving tasks | | | | |
| Helps with ADL | 2.52 (0.89) | 2.69 (0.95) | 2.09 (0.84) | 2.82 (0.91)*** |
| Helps with IADL | 3.22 (0.67) | 3.58 (0.71)*** | 2.87 (0.81) | 3.64 (0.72)*** |
| Psychosocial resources | | | | |
| Mastery | 2.44 (0.57) | 2.65 (0.60)* | 2.81 (0.61) | 2.77 (0.56) |
| Perceived support | 69.5 (22.5) | 56.5 (26.2)*** | 80.2 (22.5) | 66.8 (24.3)*** |
| Caregiving appraisal | | | | |
| Role overload | 2.75 (0.91) | 3.05 (0.85)* | 2.28 (0.86) | 2.60 (0.87)** |
| Role captivity | 2.19 (1.02) | 1.63 (0.75)*** | 1.99 (0.91) | 1.85 (0.89) |
| Positive self-esteem | 3.27 (0.58) | 3.45 (0.52)* | 3.36 (0.56) | 3.15 (0.66)** |
| Coping | | | | |
| Planful problem solving | 2.13 (0.60) | 1.78 (0.61)*** | 2.23 (0.61) | 1.92 (0.56)*** |
| Positive reappraisal | 1.41 (0.83) | 0.65 (0.63)*** | 1.30 (0.84) | 0.79 (0.69)*** |
| Seeking support | 1.77 (0.68) | 1.88 (0.59) | 2.18 (0.63) | 2.01 (0.61)* |
| Escape-avoidance | 1.33 (0.79) | 0.75 (0.50)*** | 1.27 (0.73) | 0.71 (0.56)*** |
| Distancing | 1.18 (0.83) | 1.04 (0.65) | 0.97 (0.76) | 1.07 (0.61) |
| Psychological distress | 1.02 (0.64) | 1.16 (0.66) | 0.80 (0.68) | 0.96 (0.67)* |

Notes: ADL = Activities of daily living. IADL = Instrumental ADL, SD = Standard deviation.
[a] Higher scores represent higher level of each measure. Range: ADL 0-2.2, IADL 0-1, cognitive status, psychological distress 0-4, caregiving tasks, mastery, appraisal 1-4, social support 0-100, coping 0-3.
* $P < 0.05$   ** $P < 0.01$   *** $P < 0.001$

($p = 0.06$). Similar to the findings among the spouses, the psychosocial variables accounted for most (24%) of the variance of distress.

## DISCUSSION

The major question of this study was whether culture differences explain caregiver health outcomes. Supporting Aranda and Knight (1997) argument for a sociocultural stress and coping model, the differences in psychological distress between the veteran Israeli and immigrant care-givers were mediated by the distinct caregiving stressors, appraisal, mastery and coping. These findings are consistent with the majority of previous studies concerning racial or ethnic comparisons of family caregivers (Haley et al., 1996; Knight, Silverstine, McCallum, & Fox, 2000; Patterson et al., 1998; Young & Kahana, 1995), but contradict others that found a significant direct association of ethnicity (race) with distress (Farran et al., 1997; Lawton et al., 1992; Miller et al., 1995). Additionally, the current findings, congruent with previous research (Li et al., 1997), show that caregiving stress models vary by care recipient-caregiver relationship.

It is first important to remark that even though the two groups of this study differ not only by cultural background but also by immigration sta-tus, the study design did not allow separating these two factors. However, the fact that most of the immigrant caregivers had already been living in Israel for eight to ten years allows us to conclude that the differences are mainly cultural rather than due to immigration stresses. A previous study of immigrants, up to 5 years post-immigration, showed that psychologi-cal distress, measured by the same scale as in the current study, declines with increased time living in Israel (Ritsner & Ponizovsky, 1999). The mean distress level of the immigrant caregivers in the current study (spouses and adult children together) is even lower ($1.03 \pm 0.67$) than the level for 50-69 year old immigrants, five years post immigration ($1.12 \pm 0.5$) in that study. Others have stressed the uniqueness of this immigration from the FSU that, despite an interest in acquiring the language and cul-ture of the new setting, resist total assimilation and are attached to their original culture and identity (Ben-Rafael, Olshtain, & Geijst, 1997).

Therefore, the bivariate level differences between the groups in caregiving stressors and psychosocial mediators may be interpreted by cul-tural norms and the different context of caregiving. Thus, co-residence of the elderly immigrants with their adult children (Mirsky, 1998) and the family-centered social networks (Litwin, 1995) contribute to the greater caregiving tasks of the immigrants compared to the veteran resident care-givers. Their limited social support, given that they have less supportive networks within the Israeli society (Soskolne, 2001), may be also related to the fact that they–at least among the adult children–were less likely to cope by seeking support. This may deprive them from needed additional sources of help in caregiving, further expressed in their appraisal of caregiving as being a greater role overload. Despite this, the immigrants appraised caregiving as less role-captive, possibly a reflection of the cultural norm

TABLE 3. Standardized regression coefficients (ß) in final step of hierarchical multiple regressions of psychological distress on caregiving stressors and psychosocial variables[a]

| | Spouse caregivers | Adult child caregivers |
|---|---|---|
| Group: Immigrants[b] | 0.15 | 0.07 |
| Control variables[b] | | |
| Gender: female | -- | 0.01 |
| Marital status: not married | -- | 0.05 |
| Income: < IS4500 | 0.16* | -- |
| Caregiving stressors[c] | | |
| ADL | -- | −0.16* |
| IADL | -- | -- |
| Problem behavior[b]: yes | 0.20** | 0.16** |
| Cognitive status | -- | -- |
| Helps with ADL | -- | 0.18* |
| Helps with IADL | -- | -- |
| Psychosocial resources[c] | | |
| Mastery | −0.29*** | −0.34*** |
| Caregiving appraisal | | |
| Role overload | 0.10 | 0.15* |
| Role captivity | 0.18* | 0.17* |
| Coping | | |
| Seeking support | −0.16‡ | −0.001 |
| Escape-avoidance | 0.06 | 0.12‡ |
| Distancing | −0.15* | −0.06 |
| F | 6.03*** | 8.63*** |
| DF | 12, 156 | 16, 227 |
| Adjusted R2 | 0.264 | 0.334 |

Notes: IS = Israeli shekels (4500 equivalent to $1100). ADL = Activities of daily living. IADL = Instrumental activities of daily living. DF = Degrees of freedom.
[a]Only variables significantly associated with distress at the bivariate analyses were included in the models, but perceived social support, positive self-esteem, planful problem solving, and positive reappraisal did not meet the criteria of $p < 0.10$ for entry in the final stage. [b]Dichotomous variable. [c]Continuous variables: higher scores indicate a higher level of the measure.
-- Not included, ‡ $P < 0.10$, * $P< = 0.05$, ** $P < 0.01$,  *** $P < 0.001$

that the family should carry out the bulk of eldercare (Remennick, 1999; Slonim-Nevo, Cwikel, Lusky, Lankry, & Shraga, 1995). Among the spouse caregivers, this commitment was also expressed in greater appraisal of positive aspects of caregiving than veteran Israeli spouses while the opposite direction was found among the adult child caregivers. This difference by relationship type may reflect life-course differences (Moen, Robinson, & Demster-McClain, 1995) or acculturation (Aroian, Spitzer, & Bell, 1995) that allowed the immigrant adult children to express less positive views about caregiving. While the immigrant caregivers, both spouse and adult children, resembled other minority groups in their lower use of problem and emotion-focused coping strategies (Aranda & Knight, 1997; Haley et al., 1996), the differences in psychological distress contradict the findings among other ethnic minority caregivers. Non-white caregivers–despite more difficult caregiving situations–did not differ from or reported even fewer negative psychological outcomes than White caregivers (Aranda & Knight, 1997; Dilworth-Anderson et al., 2002), but the immigrant caregivers in the current study reported higher psychological distress than the veteran Israeli caregivers. This difference is not unique to caregivers and was found in other samples of immigrants from the FSU (Mirsky, 1998; Ritsner & Ponizovsky, 1999). Yet, the non-significant difference among the spouse caregivers may be partially explained by a smaller sample size (66 immigrant spouses) or by the fact that reactions to life stress vary across the life course (Ensel, Peek, Lin, & Lai, 1996); living under chronic stress situations may reduce cultural differences in distress among the older caregivers.

The multivariate analysis supports previous caregiving research (e.g., Haley et al., 1996; Knight et al., 2000; Patterson et al., 1998; Young & Kahana, 1995) that caregiving stressors, and, to a larger extent, caregiving cognitive appraisal, psychosocial resources and coping mediate the cultural differences in psychological outcomes among the adult children. As in other studies, the presence of behavioral problems of the care recipients emerged as the main caregiving stressor and mastery as the most significant factors associated with distress in both spouse and adult child caregivers (Haley et al., 1996; Knight et al., 2000; Bookwala & Shultz, 1998; Braithwaite, 1996; Pearlin et al., 1990). Contrary to previous findings (e.g., Haley et al., 1996; Patterson et al., 1998), social support was not associated with distress. Additionally, unlike the findings of Haley et al. (1996), only emotion-focused coping strategies mediated cultural differences in psychological distress. This could be due to the greater relevance of problem-focused coping to positive mood rather than to distress (Folkman, 1997), or a result of the use of a shorter version of the coping questionnaire.

The distinct final regression models that emerged for the spouse and for the adult child caregivers imply that different factors contribute to psychological distress in each relationship type. In particular, the finding that the care recipient's problems in ADL and the caregiver's assistance with ADL were additional stressors significantly associated with psychological distress only among the adult children warrant further discussion. Others have also shown dissimilar associations of ADL to distress by relationship to care recipient (e.g., Farran et al., 1997;

Bookwala & Schulz, 1998; Young & Kahana, 1995). However, the findings in the current study among the adult child caregivers are particularly perplexing. Distress was higher when the extent of the caregiver's assistance with ADL was *greater* (as expected), yet it was also higher when the care recipient had *less* ADL limitations. This may have been a chance finding. In addition, appraisal and coping strategies associated with distress were different among the spouses and the adult child caregivers. Because previous sociocultural comparisons of family caregivers (e.g., Knight et al., 2000; Young & Kahana, 1995) did not show consistent results about the role of relationship type or age of caregivers in explaining differences in distress, further research is therefore required.

The methodology of the current study poses several limitations. The selection of participants through formal services, with no data on family caregivers who are not known to the health services, and from one metropolitan area in Israel limits representativeness. However, due to the universal provision of home aid under the Community Long-term Care Law in Israel, and the decreasing gap in use of health services between the immigrant and veteran Israelis (Habib, Noam, Elenbogen, Litvak, Naon, Nirel et al., 1998), the majority of family caregivers to patients in need of assistance in ADL or IADL are probably known to the formal services. The question whether the differences in psychosocial variables stem from cultural differences in modes of reporting, or from the fact that some of the measures–like the coping scales–were used in Russian for the first time warrants additional research. The cross-sectional design of the study limits conclusions about causality and a prospective study is recommended. Finally, since non-caregivers are not included in the current study, the differences between the groups may reflect general differences between the immigrant and the more established residents.

However, the comprehensive framework of caregiving stress of the current study contributes to the literature on family caregiving in several important ways. First, it highlights the different facets of cultural differences in caregiving stress by relationship status to the care recipient, whereas previous studies failed to do so because they either did not investigate the impact of relationship type (e.g., Haley et al., 1996; Knight et al., 2000), or studied only daughters (White et al., 2000) or spouses (Farran et al., 1997). Secondly, it showed that income, an indicator of socio-economic status thought to account for cultural differences in health outcomes (Aranda & Knight, 1997), explained psychological health only among the spouses, and with a small effect size. Third, the study population was not limited to dementia caregivers, thus allowing for greater generalization to all caregivers. Fourth, the samples of the two cultural groups were larger than many of the previous studies. Finally, the study provides a comparison in an immigrant, multi-cultural society that was not based on racial differences, responding to the need for cultural comparisons within White populations (Dilworth-Anderson et al., 2002). Therefore, the findings are relevant to other countries with immigrant populations, particularly those absorbing immigrations from Eastern Europe.

These findings have important implications for social work interventions. The structure and values of Jewish families in Israel remain relatively traditional and the majority of families still prefer to care for the disabled or ill elderly at home (Brodsky, 1998). Social workers have an important role in working with both care recipients and caregivers, given their professional training and qualifications in providing a broad and diverse scope of strategies for intervention. Such joint interventions are likely to achieve larger effects in improving caregiver burden and distress than specific narrow modes (Schultz & Martire, 2004). The current findings imply that social workers need to acquire a more refined understanding of cultural norms and the life context of the subgroups within the population. Their interventions should vary not only by immigration group but should also take into account the relationship status to the care recipient and thus be more significant in ameliorating psychological distress, particularly among immigrant adult child caregivers. Outreach programs in which Russian speaking social workers provide individual and family counseling emphasizing an intergenerational approach are recommended. Provision of additional, more flexible services at home and support groups or telephone support services in Russian may be particularly suitable interventions for these burdened immigrant caregivers.

## NOTE

1. For brevity, the term "veteran Israelis" will be used throughout the manuscript in reference to established, veteran residents in order to differentiate them from recent immigrants.

## REFERENCES

Aranda, M. P., & Knight, B. G. (1997). The influence of ethnicity and culture on the caregiver stress and coping process: A sociocultural review and analysis. *The Gerontologist, 37*, 342-354.

Aroian, K., Spitzer, A., & Bell, M. (1995). Family stress and support among former Soviet immigrants. *Western Journal of Nursing Research, 18*, 655-674.

Ben-Rafael, E., Olshtain, E., & Geijst, I. (1997). Identity and language: The social insetion of Soviet Jews in Israel. In Lewin-Epstein, N., Ro'I, Y. & Ritterband, P. (Ed.). *Russian Jews on Three Continents: Migration and Resettlement* (pp. 364-388). London: Frank Cass.

Bookwala, J., & Schulz, R. (1998). The role of neuroticism and mastery in spouse caregivers' assessment of and response to a contextual stressor. *Journal of Gerontology: Psychological Sciences, 53B*, P155-P164.

Braithwaite, V. (1996). Between stressors and outcomes: Can we simplify caregiving process variables? *The Gerontologist, 36*, 43-53.

Brodsky, J. (1998). The changing needs of the elderly in Israel and issues in the development of solutions. *Gerontology, 25*, 15-27. (Hebrew).

Brodsky, J., & Naon, D. (1993). Home care services in Israel: Implications of the expansion of home care following implementation of the Community Long-Term Care Insurance Law. *Journal of Cross-Cultural Gerontology, 8*, 375-390.

Cohen, J., & Cohen, P. (1983). Applied Multiple Regression/Correlation Analysis for Behavioral Sciences (2nd ed.). Hillsdale, NJ: Elbaum.

Dilworth-Anderson, P., Williams, I. C., & Gibson, B. E. (2002). Issues of race, ethnicity, and culture in caregiving research: A 20-year review (1980-2000). *The Gerontologist, 42*, 237-272.

Ensel, W. M., Peek, M. K., Lin, N., & Lai, G. (1996). Stress in the life course: A life history approach. *Journal of Aging and Health, 8*, 389-416.

Farran, C. J., Miller, B. H., Kaufman, J. E., & Davis, L. (1997). Race, finding meaning, and caregiver distress. *Journal of Aging and Health, 9*, 316-333.

Fillenbaum, G. (1985). Screening the elderly: A brief Instrumental Activities of Daily Living measure. *Journal of the American Geriatric Society, 33*, 698-706.

Folkman, S. (1997). Positive psychological states and coping with severe stress. *Social Science and Medicine, 45*, 1207-1221.

Folkman, S., Lazarus, R. S., Pimley, S., & Novacek, J. (1987). Age differences in stress and coping processes. *Psychology and Aging, 2*, 171-184.

Habib, J., Noam, G., Elenbogen, S., Litvak, I., Naon, D., Nirel, N., Strosberg, N., & Beer, S. (1998). Risk groups among the immigrants. In M. Sicron & E. Leshem (Eds.), *Profile of an immigration wave* (pp. 409-441). Jerusalem: Magnes, The Hebrew University. (Hebrew).

Haley, W. E., Roth, D. L., Coleton, M. I., Ford, G. R., West, C. A. C., Collins, R. P., & Isobe, T. L. (1996). Appraisal, coping, and social support as mediators of well-being in Black and White family caregivers of patients with Alzheimer's disease. *Journal of Consulting and Clinical Psychology, 64*, 121-129.

Idler, E. I., & Benyamini, Y. (1997). Self-rated health and mortality: A review of twenty community studies. *Journal of Health and Social Behavior, 38*, 21-37.

Knight, B. G., Silverstein, M., McCallum, T. J., & Fox, L. S. (2000). A sociocultural stress and coping model for mental health outcomes among African American caregivers in Southern California. *Journal of Gerontology: Psychological Sciences, 55B*, P142-P150.

Kulik, L. (2001). Attitudes toward spousal caregiving and their correlates among aging women. *Journal of Women & Aging, 13,* 41-58.

Lawton, M. P., Rajagopal, D., Brody, E., & Kleban, M. H. (1992). The dynamics of caregiving for a demented elder among Black and White families. *Journal of Gerontology: Social Sciences, 47,* S156-S164.

Lazarus, R. S., & Folkman, S. (1984). *Stress, appraisal and coping.* New York: Springer Publishing Company.

Li, W. L., Seltzer M. M., & Greenberg, J. S. (1997). Social support and depressive symptoms: Differential patterns in wife and daughter caregivers. *Journal of Gerontology: Social Sciences, 52B,* S200-S211.

Litwin, H. (1994). Filial responsibility and informal support among family caregivers of the elderly in Jerusalem: A path analysis. *International Journal of Aging and Human Development, 38,* 137-151.

Litwin, H. (1995). *Uprooted in old age: Soviet Jews and their social networks in Israel.* Westport, CT: Greenwood Press.

Manor, O., Power, C., and Matthews, S. (2001). Self rated health and limiting long-standing illness: Inter-relationships with morbidity in early adulthood. *International Journal of Epidemiology, 30,* 600-607.

Miller, B. H., Campbell, R. T., Farran, C. J., Kaufman, J. E., & Davis, L. (1995). Race, control, mastery, and caregiver distress. *Journal of Gerontology: Social Sciences, 50B,* S374-S382.

Mirsky, J. (1998). Psychological aspects in immigration and absorption of immigrants from the Soviet Union. In M. Sicron & E. Leshem (Eds.), *Profile of an immigration wave* (pp. 334-367). Jerusalem: Magnes, The Hebrew University. (Hebrew).

Moen, P., Robinson, J., & Demster-McClain, D. (1995). Caregiving and women's well-being: A life course approach. *Journal of Health and Social Behavior, 36,* 259-273.

Moskowitz-Tedlie, J., Folkman, S., Collette, L., & Vittinghoff, E. (1996). Coping and mood during AIDS-related caregiving and bereavement. *Annals of Behavioral Medicine, 18,* 49-57.

Nijboer, C., Triemstra, M., Tempelaar, R., Sanderman, R., & van den Bos, G. A. M. (1999). Measuring both negative and positive reactions to giving care to cancer patients: Psychometric qualities of the Caregiver Reaction Assessment (CRA). *Social Science and Medicine, 48,* 1259-1269.

Nirel, N., Rosen, B., Gross, R., Berg, A., & Youval, D. (1996). *Immigrants from the Former Soviet Union in the health system: Selected findings from national surveys.* JDC-Brookdale Institute, Jerusalem, Israel. (Hebrew).

Noonan, A. E., & Tennstedt, S. (1997). Meaning in caregiving and its contribution to caregiver well-being. *The Gerontologist, 37,* 785-794.

Patterson, T. L., Semple, S. J., Shaw, W. S., Yu, E., He, Y., Zhang, M. Y., Wu, W., & Grant, I. (1998). The cultural context of caregiving: A comparison of Alzheimer's caregivers in Shanghai, China and San Diego, California. *Psychological Medicine, 28,* 1071-1084.

Pearlin, L. I., Mullan, J. T., Semple, S. J., & Skaff, M. M. (1990). Caregiving and the stress process: An overview of concepts and their measures. *The Gerontologist, 30,* 583-594.

Pearlin, L. I., & Schooler, C. (1978). The structure of coping. *Journal of Health and Social Behavior, 19*, 2-21.

Pot, A. M., Deeg, D. J. H., van Dyck, R., & Jonker, C. (1998). Psychological distress of caregivers: The mediator effect of caregiving appraisal. *Patient Education and Counseling, 34*, 43-51.

Remennick, L. I. (1999). Women of the "sandwich" generation and multiple roles: The case of Russian immigrants of the 1990s in Israel. *Sex Roles, 40*, 347-378.

Remennick, L. I. (2001). "All my life is one big nursing home": Russian immigrant women in Israel speak about double caregiver stress. *Women's Studies International Forum, 24*, 685-700.

Ritsner, M., Rabinowitz, J., & Slyuzberg, M. (1995). The Talbieh Brief Distress Inventory: A brief instrument to measure psychological distress among immigrants. *Comprehensive Psychiatry, 36*, 448-453.

Ritsner, M., & Ponizovsky, A. (1999). The Psychological distress through immigration. The two-phase temporal pattern? *International Journal of Social Psychiatry, 45*, 125-139.

Ritsner M., & Ponizovsky, A. (2003). Age differences in stress process of recent immigrants. *Comprehensive Psychiatry, 44*, 135-141.

Schulz, R., & Martire, L. M. (2004). Family caregiving of persons with dementia: Prevalence, health effects, and support strategies. *American Journal of Geriatric Psychiatry, 12*, 240-249.

Sherbourne Donald, C., & Stewart, A. L. (1991). The MOS Social Support Survey. *Social Science and Medicine, 32*, 705-714.

Slonim-Nevo, V., Cwikel, J., Lusky, H., Lankry, M., & Shraga, Y. (1995). Caregiver burden among three-generation immigrant families in Israel. *International Social Work, 38*, 191-204.

Soskolne, V. (2001). Single parenthood, occupational drift and psychological distress among immigrant women from the former Soviet Union in Israel. *Women & Health, 33*, 67-84.

Strosberg, N., & Naon, D. (1997). Older Immigrants from the Former Soviet Union: Follow-up of Absorption in Housing and Other Areas for the Years 1992-1995. JDC-Brookdale Institute, Jerusalem, Israel.

Tennstedt, S. (1999). Family Caregiving in an Aging Society. Presented at the U.S. Administration on Aging Symposium: Longevity in the New American Century, Baltimore, March 29, 1999.

Thoits, P. A. (1995). Stress, coping, and social support processes: Where are we? What next? *Journal of Health and Social Behavior, 36* (Extra Issue), 53-79.

Walter-Ginzburg, A., Guralnik, J. M., Blumstein, T., Gindin, J., & Modan, B. (2001). Assistance with personal care activities among the old-old in Israel: A national epidemiological study. *Journal of the American Geriatric Society, 49*, 1176-1184.

White, T. M., Townsend, A. L., & Stephens Parris, M. A. (2000). Comparisons of African American and White women in the parent care role. *The Gerontologist, 40*, 718-728.

Yates, M. E., Tennstedt, S., & Chang, B.-H. (1999). Contributors to and mediators of psychological well-being for informal caregivers. *Journal of Gerontology: Psychological Sciences, 54B*, P12-P22.

Youn, G., Knight, B. G., Jeong, H., & Benton, D. (1999). Differences in familism values and caregiving outcomes among Korean, Korean American, and White American caregivers. *Psychology and Aging, 14*, 355-364.

Young, R. F., & Kahana, E. (1995). The context of caregiving and well-being outcomes among African and Caucasian Americans. *The Gerontologist, 35*, 225-232.

# When Disaster Becomes Commonplace: Reaction of Children and Adolescents to Prolonged Terrorist Attacks in Israel

Shlomo A. Sharlin, PhD
Victor Moin, PhD
Rivka Yahav, PhD

**SUMMARY.** The aim of this study was to examine, in conditions of prolonged terror, the possible influences of yet another terrorist attack as an additional traumatic event on children's reactions in the emotional, behavioral, and cognitive spheres, and to identify any mediating factors. The sample included 747 students in junior high schools in three Israeli cities. None of the participants were directly exposed to terrorist attacks, but they all lived with the possibility of daily terror. The research focused on fear as the most common and widespread reaction to terror and war. Short-term and long-term symptoms of fear were studied. It was found that an additional terrorist attack had no significant influence on

Shlomo A. Sharlin is Professor, Victor Moin is Senior Researcher, and Rivka Yahav is Senior Lecturer The Center for Research and Study of the Family, Faculty of Social Welfare and Health Studies, University of Haifa.

Address correspondence to: Shlomo A. Sharlin, PhD, The Center for Research and Study of the Family, Faculty of Social Welfare and Health Studies, University of Haifa, Mount Carmel, Haifa 31905, Israel (E-mail: moin@research.haifa.ac.il, sharlin@research. haifa.ac.il).

[Haworth co-indexing entry note]: "When Disaster Becomes Commonplace: Reaction of Children and Adolescents to Prolonged Terrorist Attacks in Israel." Sharlin, Shlomo A.,Victor Moin, and Rivka Yahav. Co-published simultaneously in *Social Work in Health Care* (The Haworth Press, Inc.) Vol. 43, No. 2/3, 2006, pp. 95-114; and: *International Social Health Care Policy, Programs, and Studies* (ed: Gary Rosenberg, and Andrew Weissman) The Haworth Press, Inc., 2006, pp. 95-114. Single or multiple copies of this article are available for a fee from The Haworth Document Delivery Service [1-800-HAWORTH, 9:00 a.m. - 5:00 p.m. (EST). E-mail address: docdelivery@haworthpress.com].

Available online at http://swhc.haworthpress.com
© 2006 by The Haworth Press, Inc. All rights reserved.
doi:10.1300/J010v43n02_07

children's emotional, cognitive, or behavioral spheres. Terror that has become habitual becomes negligible. Children learn to adjust to loss without experiencing grief. *[Article copies available for a fee from The Haworth Document Delivery Service: 1-800-HAWORTH. E-mail address: <docdelivery@haworthpress.com> Website: <http://www.HaworthPress.com> © 2006 by The Haworth Press, Inc. All rights reserved.]*

**KEYWORDS.** Terror, children, adolescents, fear

## INTRODUCTION

The aim of this study was to examine, in conditions of prolonged terror, the possible influences of yet another terrorist attack as an additional traumatic event on children's reactions in the emotional, behavioral, and cognitive spheres, and to identify any mediating factors.

War and terrorist attacks are considered among the most painful and traumatic events. They erode the sense of security and give rise to fear, anxiety, depression, mental disorders and behavioral problems (e.g., Barenbaum, Ruchkin, & Schwab-Stone, 2004; Bleich, Gelkopf, & Solomon, 2003; Galea, & Resnick, 2005; North, Nixon, Shariat, Mallonee, McMillen, Spitzanagel, & Smith, 1999; Smith, Christiansen, Vincent, & Hann, 1999; Schuster, Stein, Jaycox, Collins, Marshall, Elliott, Zhou, Kanouse, Morrison, & Berry, 2001; Schlenger, Caddell, Ebert, Jordan, Rourke, Wilson, Thalji, Dennis, Fairbank, & Kulka, 2002).

Most studies on the consequences of child exposure to terrorism focus on the stressful effects of isolated and sudden terrorist attacks (e.g., the Oklahoma City bombing, 1993; events of September 11, 2001) and on the people directly exposed to them (Barenbaum, Ruchkin, & Schwab-Stone, 2004; Bleich, Gelkopf, & Solomon, 2003). However, the stressful nature of a sudden isolated terrorist attack differs qualitatively from that of recurrent, chronic terror. According to Terr (1991), there are two types of trauma: Type 1 trauma produces Post-Traumatic Stress Disorder (PTSD) symptoms after a one-time sudden traumatic event; Type 2 trauma is the result of long-term repeated exposure to trauma. The former cause significant stressful effects (Desivilya, Gal, & Ayalon, 1996; Koplewicz, Vogel, Solanto, Morrissey, Alonso, Abikoff, Gallagher, & Novick, 2002; North et al., 1999; Smith et al., 1999; Schuster et al., 2001; Schlenger et al., 2002). After mass terrorist incidents, there may be posttraumatic stress symptoms not only among those directly exposed to the attack, but also among those in the general population who were not directly exposed to the attacks (Galea & Resnick, 2005). By contrast, war and prolonged terror do not always lead to mental and behavioral problems (e.g., Barenbaum, Ruchkin, & Schwab-Stone, 2004; Weisaeth, 1997; Zeidner, 1993).

In Israel, children and adolescents live in conditions of prolonged terror most all their lives. In 1987, Palestinians began their uprising in the West Bank and the Gaza Strip, known as the first Intifada. In October 2000, the second Intifada began, and it is still in effect. Suicide bombers have exploded in many of the cities of Israel. Since this uprising began, over four years ago, it has claimed the lives of thousands of men, women, and children and has wounded thousands of civilians, on both sides.

However, even in conditions of prolonged terror in such a small country as Israel, the majority of the population is not directly exposed to terrorist attacks. According to a nationally representative sample taken in Israel, only 16.4% of the 512 surveyed participants had been directly exposed to terrorist attacks (Bleich, Gelkopf, & Solomon, 2003). The object of our study is to observe the reactions of children and adolescents who were not directly exposed to terrorist attacks but who live in conditions of prolonged terror in Israel.

The extent of stress experienced after a disaster varies as a function of a wide variety of factors. These include the overall socio-cultural and political context (Shamai, 2002; Solomon & Lavi, 1999; Weisaeth, 1997; Tobin, 2000); media involvement (Keinan, Sadeh, & Rosen, 2003; Ryan-Wenger, 2001; Schlenger et al., 2002; Zeidner, 1993; Slone, 2000); close network, family and friends (Koplewicz et al., 2002; Jones, Ribbe, & Cunningham, 1994; Shamai, 2002); personal factors, in particular the level of social-emotional and cognitive development (Joshi, & O'Donnell, 2003); and situational factors directly related to the traumatic event (e.g., Barenbaum, Ruchkin, & Schwab-Stone, 2004; Joshi, & O'Donnell, 2003; Koplewicz et al., 2002; Zeidner, 1993).

We studied four group factors that affected children's reactions to the new terrorist attack: (1) situational factors and their potential traumatic effect (level of disruption as a consequence of the terrorist attack, its geographical location, and length of time elapsed after the attack); (2) close network (perceived reactions of parents and friends to terrorist acts); (3) children and parents' concentration on the media; (4) children's characteristics (gender, age, and behavioral problems, including aggression, delinquency, attention disorder, thinking disorder, depression, social problems, anxiety, and regressive behavior).

War and terror are a complex mixture of psychologically traumatic events. Their impact is wide-ranging and multi-faceted and it may affect all areas of personality. (See reviews, Barenbaum, Ruchkin, & Schwab-Stone, 2004; Joshi, & O'Donnell, 2003.) In the emotional sphere its most common and conspicuous expressions are Posttraumatic Stress Disorder (PTSD), depression, fear, and anxiety. In the cognitive sphere, there is damage to concentration, memory, and learning abilities (Girdon, 2002). In the behavioral sphere, social, family, and occupational functioning may be compromised (Solomon & Lavi, 1999).

To study the reactions of non-exposed children and adolescents to a terrorist attack in conditions of prolonged terror, the research focused on fear as the most common and widespread reaction to terror and war (Muris, Meesters, Mayer, Bogie, Luijten, Geebelen, Bessems, & Smit, 2003; Muris & Ollendick, 2002; Shamai, 2002; Walter, 2002).

Fear is one of the significant stress symptoms. "Fear has the potential and capacity to paralyze children and negatively impact their emotional growth" (Joshi & O'Donnell, 2003, p. 280). It manifests itself in various actions, reflections, attitudes, and feelings. It can be expressed as nervousness, trauma, agitation, tension, stress, restlessness, sleep problems, or inability to cope with ordinary life issues.

As far as we can ascertain, most frequently used methods measuring children's fears (Ollendick, 1983; McCathie & Spence, 1991; Muris, Merckelbach, Ollendick, King, Meestrs, & van Kessel, 2002; Muris et al., 2003) address mainly the intensity of object-oriented fears. The instruments just listed do not analyze the various spheres of fear manifestation. Our main focus in this study is on self-reported manifestations of fear of terrorist attacks, in various domains: (a) in the emotional-cognitive domain as acknowledgment and cognitive acceptance of the danger of death in conditions of daily terror; (b) in the emotional-behavioral sphere, avoidance of specific, concrete forms of everyday activity; (c) in the cognitive-behavioral, as a fixation of mind and behavior on the object of fear (everyday thought and talk about terror and listening a great deal to the news), and (d) in the cognitive domain, the child's weakened concentration and learning ability.

This paper focuses on the following research questions: (1) Does life in conditions of prolonged terror lead to pathological behavior problems among non-exposed children? (2) What is the intensity and prevalence of school children's fear of terrorist attacks in conditions of daily terror in Israel? Does long-term real danger lead to increased intensity of children's fears, mental and behavioral problems? (3) What are the similarities and differences between the numerous reactions to daily terror in the various spheres of a child's personality? (4) What is the effect of a new terrorist attack as an additional traumatic event on children's fears? Has this latest attack produced additional fears in children? What is the role of situational factors in the level of disruption, time scope, and the child's place of residence? (5) How does children's own fear of terror relate to the perception of parents' and friends' fears?

## *METHOD*

### *Participants and Procedure*

The sample includes 747 participants. All participants are students aged 11 to 15: 53% of them are elementary school children, 11 or 12 years old, and 47% are adolescents, 13 to 15 years old. In this paper, the term "children" will be used to indicate both groups of participants, children and adolescents. Boys account for 45% of the participants.

It is well known that reaction to war and terrorism typically varies by age and gender: girls report greater fear than do boys, while adolescents tend to experience more traumas than do children (e.g., Josi & O'Donnell, 2003; Ryan-Wenger, 2001; Weisaeth, 1997). These tendencies were also found in this study. Though age and gender differences in their reaction to terror were not the object of special attention in this paper, these variables were included in a regression analysis and structural equation models.

All participants were non-exposed children: none of them had been a direct witness or a victim of the terrorist attack, nor had any of their relatives or friends. The participants lived in Haifa, a city in northern Israel, in Ariel, a Jewish city in the Samaria (West Bank) region, and in Jerusalem. Data were collected after three terrorist attacks:

(1) In *Haifa, 4 April 2002.* The suicide bomber arrived at the Matza Restaurant while the place was full of diners. Ironically, this restaurant is owned by Jews and Arabs and serves as an example of peaceful co-existence. Fourteen people were killed, several among them were Arabs; 39 people were wounded.
(2) In *Ariel, 18 October 2002.* The suicide bomber arrived at a parking area next to a gas station. He was identified and soldiers tried to disarm him. However, their attempts failed and the terrorist managed to blow himself up. Three people were killed and 20 wounded.

(3) In *Jerusalem, 22 November 2002*. Jerusalem's bus #20 exploded after a suicide bomber got on. The bus, which serves the residential areas, was full of children on their way to school. Eleven people were killed and 50 wounded.

Data were collected at various points in time, shortly after and a month following each of these terrorist attacks. Data were also obtained from different cities where an attack occurred, and from a control city that had not suffered an attack.

### *Instruments*

Two main instruments were used to measure research variables: (1) Children's Reaction to Terror Questionnaire (CRTQ); and (2) Child Behavioral Checklist (CBCL)–Youth Self Report (YSR; Achenbach and Edelbrock, 1987).

*Children's Reaction to Terror Questionnaire (CRTQ)* was constructed specifically for this study. The CRTQ consisted of 22 items. The children were asked to rate to what degree each statement correctly reflected his or her feeling on a five-point scale ranging from 1, "Absolutely wrong," to 5, "Absolutely right." The CRTQ measured reactions to terror in different areas of personality: emotional-cognitive (general fear); emotional-behavioral (fear of everyday activity); behavioral (preoccupation), cognitive (concentration and learning ability). It also measured the network context: perception of parents' and friends' reactions to terrorist attacks.

*Children's reactions to terror* were measured by four variables: Child's General Fear Scale (CGFS), Child's Everyday Fear Scale (CEFS), Child's Preoccupation Scale (CPS), and Child's Weakening Concentration (CWC). Each of these variables was characterized by two parameters: prevalence rate, i.e., percentage of children experiencing fear, and intensity of fear, assessed by the rating indicated on a five-point scale.

General fear of terror attacks was conceptualized as acknowledgment, cognitive acceptance, and awareness of the danger of death in conditions of daily terror. General fear characterizes the emotional-cognitive reactions to terror. Being afraid means knowing, understanding and realizing the real dangers of life. *Child's General Fear Scale (CGFS)* was calculated as the mean of three items: "I fear suicide terrorists," "I fear being hurt in terrorist attacks," and "I worry about the security situation in Israel" (Cronbach's alpha = .80).

In the emotional-behavioral sphere, everyday fears were defined as an avoidance of specific, concrete forms of everyday activity. Being afraid means avoidance of activities because of the danger they may involve. For example, in Israel there is the fear of traveling by bus, of going to a mall, or sitting in restaurants and coffee-shops. *Child's Everyday Fear Scale* (CEFS) was calculated as the mean of six items: "I fear riding a bus," "I fear going to a mall," "I fear going to the movies," "I fear sitting in restaurants or coffee-shops," "I fear going to the beach," and "I fear going on trips" (Cronbach's alpha = .82).

Fear as a preoccupation was conceptualized as a fixation of mind and behavior on the object of fear (everyday thought, talking about terror, listening a great deal to the news). *Child's Preoccupation Scale (CPS)* was calculated as the mean of four items: "Every day I think of a possible terror attack," "I talk to my friends about the security situation," "We talk at home about the security situation," and "I listen a great deal to the news" (Cronbach's alpha = .75).

*Child's Weakened Concentration (CWC)*. The impact of terrorist acts on the cognitive domain was measured by one item: "The security situation has a bad influence on my ability to concentrate on my studies."

*Family context* was characterized by the child's perception of his or her parents' reactions to terror: the parents' general anxiety scale (emotional reactions), parents' control of the child's behavior (behavioral reactions) and parents' informative loading (cognitive-behavioral sphere).

*Parents' Anxiety Scale (PAS)* was calculated as the mean of two items: "My mother worries about the security situation in Israel," "My father worries about the security situation in Israel" (Cronbach's alpha = .81). *Parents' Control Scale (PCS)* was calculated as the mean of two items: "My mother restrains me because of the security situation in Israel," "My father restrains me because of the security situation in Israel" (Cronbach's alpha = .83). *Parents' Informative Loading Scale (PILS)* was calculated as the mean of two items: "My mother listens to the news over the media a great deal," and "My father listens to the news over the media a great deal" (Cronbach's alpha = .75). The perception of friends' reactions to terror acts (friends' fear) was measured by one question: "My friends are afraid of terrorism."

*Child Behavioral Checklist (CBCL)*–The Youth Self Report (YSR), which was developed by Achenbach and Edelbrock (1987), presents various behavioral problems ranging from normal to pathological. Two major aspects are tested: one is competence vs. weakness in the areas of school achievements, interpersonal relationships, leisure activities, creativity, and voluntary activities. The second aspect encompasses eight different subgroups of behavior problems, specifically: aggression, delinquency, attention disorder, thinking disorder, depression, social problems, anxiety, and regressive behavior. Responses are rated on a five-point scale. The validity of the scale was tested in a test-retest study over a period of one week, with the result of r = .81. The Hebrew version was developed by the Falk Institute in 1989 and the Israeli norms were matched. The reliability of the Hebrew version was assessed by Cronbach's alpha, which was found to be .92 (.93 in our study).

*Situational factors* included the following variables: level of disruption as a consequence of the terrorist attack, its location, and the time that elapsed since the attack. *Level of disruption*, determined according to the number of victims, was identified in this study as "Severe" in Ariel, and "Very Severe" in Haifa and Jerusalem. Two groups of children were identified according to *geographical location*: children living in the city where the terrorist attack occurred and children living in other cities. Two groups were identified in regard to *time elapsed*: children who were interviewed shortly after the terrorist attack and those interviewed within a month following the terrorist acts.

These situational variables were factors in considering the potential traumatic effect of terrorist attacks on children. Thus, it was assumed that the potential traumatic effect of a terrorist attack with a high number of victims would be stronger shortly after the occurrence rather than a month later, and similarly, that the traumatic effect would be stronger on children living in the city where the attack occurred compared to the effect on those living in other cities. Accordingly, the general indicator of Potential Traumatic Effect (PTE) of terrorist attacks was measured as accumulative variables–the sum of the situational variables.

## RESULTS

Life in conditions of prolonged terror does not lead to pathological behavior problems among non-exposed children (according to Achenbach's Child Behavioral Checklist). In our study, the prevalence rate and intensity of fear were found to be relatively low. Reactions to terror are different in various spheres of personality: most children understood the dangers to terror, yet they were not overly preoccupied by this; they behaved quite bravely in their everyday activities. High internal consistency was found to exist between reactions to terror in various spheres of personality. Nevertheless, there were also significant differences between reactions in terms of their intensity and the factors determining various reactions. A new terrorist attack did not produce significant additional fears in children. The place of residence, belonging to the community where the terrorist attack occurred, the level of disruption, and the time scope did not impact children's reactions, in most cases. Terror that has become habitual becomes commonplace.

### Children's Behavioral Problems

There were no pathological behavior problems among children in our samples. The mean score for each area with behavioral problems, as well as the total score for behavioral problems, was far below the borderline clinical range. For example, the total score for behavioral problems in our sample was 32.8 as compared to 67-70 for borderline clinical range; for attention problems, 8.3 compared to 18-21, respectively; thought problems, 2.6 to 7-8; social problems, 2.8 to 7-8; and aggression, 8.3 to 18-21. Also, there were no significant differences between children in Haifa and Ariel in the level of behavioral problems. The total score for behavioral problems for students in Haifa was 30.9 as compared to 33.5 in Ariel.

### Prevalence Rate and Intensity of Fear

The prevalence rate and intensity of fear were found to be relatively low in the various spheres of personality:

In the *emotional-cognitive* Child's General Fear Scale–(CGFS), most children acknowledged the danger of a new terrorist attack. Prevalence rate of fear was relatively high: 64% of children were afraid "of suicide bombers," 64% "worr[ied] about the security situation in Israel," and 58% were afraid "of being injured by shooting." However, the percentage of children extremely afraid ("very" or "very much") was relatively small, from 10% to 19%. Overall, the index for general fear intensity in the emotional-cognitive sphere was low 2.19 (SD = .98).

In the *emotional-behavioral* sphere, children behaved quite bravely in their daily activities (Child's Everyday Fear Scale–CEFS). They did not avoid the more dangerous forms of everyday activity. Most of the children reported that they absolutely did not fear riding a bus (75%), going to the mall (89%), coffee shops (85%), the movies (94%), the beach (93%), and on trips (86%). Prevalence rates of fear were 25%, 11%, 15%, 6%, 7%, and 14%, respectively. The degree of intensity of everyday fear was also very low. Only 1%-2% of children feared ("very" or "very much") terror in their everyday activities. Index of intensity was only 1.18 (SD = .32).

In the *behavioral sphere*, children were not over-preoccupied with the danger. They did not think about terrorism: 72% "absolutely not," and only 5% thought about terrorism "much" or "very much." They did not listen to media news: 58% "absolutely not," and only 5% listened very, and very much. They did not talk to their friends about terrorism: 70% "absolutely not," only 5% talked a great deal. They did not talk at home about the security situation: 50% "absolutely not," 27% "not much." The index of intensity of Child's Preoccupation Scale was very low (1.6). Terrorism did not impact on the process of learning: "absolutely" (88%) and only 2% of the children marked "very" and "very much" weakened concentration.

### Children's Reaction to Terror in the Various Spheres of Personality

High internal consistency was found to exist between reactions to terror in various spheres of personality: emotional-cognitive (CGFS); emotional-behavior (CEFS); behavioral (CPS) and cognitive (CWC). The mean correlation among the four was r = .44, p < .001. Only one factor was extracted in the factor analysis (the Principal component method, rotation Varimax) from these various aspects of reaction to terror. Nevertheless, there were also significant differences between reactions, in terms of their intensity and the factors determining various reactions. In all these cases, differences between indicators of fear manifestations in the various spheres were significant, according to paired t-test (see Table 1).

Reactions in the *emotional-cognitive* sphere (Child General Fear Scale) were found to be more intense than reactions in other spheres, according to paired-samples t-testing (see Table 1). The variance in CGFS can be explained by examining the close network context: parent anxiety, friend anxiety, and parent informative loading (see results of multiple regression analysis, Table 2). Situational factors (PTE of the new terrorist attack) in no way explained the variance in CGFS.

Reactions in *the emotional-behavioral* (Child Everyday Fear Scale) were less intense than in other spheres. The index of CEFS was lower

TABLE 1. Correlation and paired t-test for child reaction to terror (N = 747)

| Pair | Variables | M | SD | Correlation | t |
|------|-----------|-----|-----|-------------|------|
| 1 | General Fear | 2.19 | .96 | | |
| | Everyday Fear | 1.18 | .38 | .44*** | 31.8*** |
| 2 | General Fear | 2.19 | .96 | | |
| | Preoccupation | 1.6 | .70 | .50*** | 18.5*** |
| 3 | General Fear | 2.19 | .96 | | |
| | Weakening of Concentration | 1.21 | .65 | .33*** | 27.3*** |
| 4 | Everyday Fear | 1.18 | .38 | | |
| | Preoccupation | 1.6 | .70 | .45*** | 17.9*** |
| 5 | Everyday Fear | 1.18 | .38 | | |
| | Weakening of Concentration | 1.21 | .65 | .43*** | 1.4 |
| 6 | Preoccupation | 1.6 | .70 | | |
| | Weakening of Concentration | 1.21 | .65 | .46*** | 14.8*** |

*** $p < .001$

than the indexes of CGFS and CPS and it was similar to index of CWC (see Table 1). According to multiple regression analysis, variances in CEFS were explained by other variables (than CGFS): mainly by parental control and situational factors–Potential Traumatic Effect (PTE) of the new terrorist attack (see Table 2).

Reactions in *the behavioral-cognitive sphere* (Child Preoccupation Scale) were less intense than in the emotional-cognitive, but they were more intense than in the emotional-behavior and cognitive spheres (see Table 1). Variance in CPS was explained by both network context (friend anxiety, parent anxiety, parent informative loading) and the additional traumatic event, as revealed in Table 2.

*In the cognitive sphere*, the weakened ability of children to concentrate was found to be very small. The variance of weakened concentration was explained mainly by situational factors (PTE of the new terrorist attack) and parental control (see Table 2).

## Traumatic Effect of a New Terrorist Attack

Each new terrorist attack is an additional traumatic event. Its Potential Traumatic Effect (PTE) is analyzed as a function of the level of disruption following the attack, its geographical location, and length of time elapsed after the attack. A few hypotheses have been posited in regard to the links between these situational factors and the reactions of

TABLE 2. Results of multiple regression analysis for children's reactions to terror in the various spheres of personality (Standardized $\beta^2$)

| Variables | General fear | Everyday fear | Preoccupation | Weakening of Concentration |
|---|---|---|---|---|
| Age | .06 | .10** | .13*** | .11*** |
| Gender | .15*** | .10** | −.10*** | .04 |
| Parent Anxiety | .29*** | .08 | .21*** | .10* |
| Parent Control | .01 | .27*** | .09** | .21*** |
| Parent Informative Loading | .17*** | .09* | .20*** | .08 |
| Friend Anxiety | .24*** | .17*** | .25*** | .15*** |
| Additional Traumatic Event | .06 | .22*** | .21*** | .27*** |
| $R^2$ | .40 | .29 | .42 | .27 |
| F | 60.8*** | 36.1*** | 88.0*** | 32.8*** |

* p < .05, ** p < .01, *** p < .001

children to daily terror: (1) Reaction of non-exposed children to the next terrorist attack will be much stronger in the community where the terrorist attack occurs; (2) Symptoms of distress are more intense shortly after the terrorist attack than after a month; and (3) The more dramatic the disruption after a terrorist attack, the stronger the reaction of children to an attack.

The research data did not support the main part of these hypotheses, or they support them only partially. Findings are reported respectively.

(1) Reaction of children to another terrorist attack was not much stronger in the community where the terrorist attack occurred. Statistically significant differences were found only in one case: fear of everyday activity was somewhat higher in the community where the terrorist attack occurred than in the community where there was no attack (index CEFS = 1.15 vs. 1.09, F = 4.04, p = .036).

(2) Time scope impacted the reaction of children in three cases: indexes of CEFS, CPS, and CWC were found to be somewhat higher shortly after the terrorist attack than in the month following the attack (CEFS = 1.3 vs. 1.1, f = 17.3, p = .001; CPS = 1.8 vs. 1.5, f = 26, p = .001; CWC = 1.4 vs. 1.1, f = 26, p = .001). However, these differences were also very small.

(3) The hypothesis that the more dramatic the disruption following a terrorist attack the stronger the children's reaction would be to this attack was also not supported by our results. Differences between reactions of children to terrorist attacks in Haifa (2002) and in Ariel were

not even in one case statistically significant (according to a post-hoc comparison, Scheffe), although the disruptions due to these attacks were very significant.

Thus, according to our findings, the situational factors related to recurring terrorist attacks did not influence the reaction of children. Belonging to the community where the terrorist attack occurred, the level of disruption, and the time scope, in most cases did not impact children's reactions. The traumatic effect of a new terrorist attack on non-exposed children was minimal. These attacks did not produce significant additional fears in children.

## Children's Perception of Their Parents' Reactions to Terror

Children attributed to their parents a higher intensity and greater prevalence of fear related to terror than to themselves. In all cases, differences were statistically significant according to Paired Samples Test as revealed in Table 3.

In all studies reviewed, children's responses to disaster were associated with those of their parents (Koplewicz et al., 2002; Jones, Ribbe & Cunningham, 1994; Shamai, 2002). Family resilience is analyzed as a mediator between the traumatic event and its impact on family members. However, in most of these studies, the children and/or their parents underwent direct disaster exposure (Koplewicz et al., 2002). It is unclear how children's reactions associate with those of their parents when neither the children nor the parents have been directly exposed to a traumatic event.

We focused on the examination of two hypotheses regarding the link between children's responses to a new terrorist attack and children's perception of their parents' and friends' reactions: (1) The mediating hypothesis assumed that the additional terrorist attack affects reactions of children mainly through perception of the reactions of close social environment (parents and friends). (2) The projection hypothesis states that children project their reactions to terrorist attacks onto their parents and friends, attributing their own fears and attitudes to their parents and friends.

To examine these hypotheses, we analyzed unrecursive structural equation models (see Figure 1). The models included the same variables: two latent variables (Child's Reactions to Terror (CRT), Parents' Reactions to Terror–PRT), four observers-related variables (age, gender, Friends' Reactions to Terror, and *Potential Traumatic Effect (PTE)*

TABLE 3. Correlation and paired t-test for child and perceived parent reaction to terror (N = 747)

| Pair | Variables | M | SD | Correlation | t |
|------|-----------|---|----|-----------|---|
| 1 | Parents General Anxiety | 2.3 | 1.1 | | |
| | Child General Fear | 2.19 | .96 | .53*** | 3.1** |
| 2 | Parents Informative Loading | 2.6 | 1.0 | | |
| | Child Preoccupation | 1.6 | .70 | .49*** | 29.6*** |
| 3 | Parents Control | 1.5 | .81 | | |
| | Child Everyday Fear | 1.18 | .38 | .40*** | 12.7*** |
| 4 | Friends General Fear | 1.6 | .92 | | |
| | Child General Fear | 2.19 | .96 | .46*** | −14.9*** |

** p < .01, *** p < .001

FIGURE 1. Unrecusive structural equation models

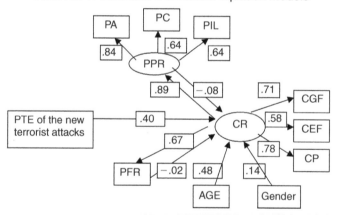

Notes:
**PTE**–Potential Traumatic Effect of the new terrorist attacks (situation factor).
**PPR**–Perceived Parents Reactions to the new terrorist attacks: **PA**–parents' anxiety; **PC**–parents' control; **PIL**–Parents' Informative Loading. **PFR**–Perceived Friends Reactions to the new terrorist attacks. **CR**–reported Child's Reactions to the new terrorist attacks: **CGF**–Child's General Fear; **CEF**–Child's Everyday Fear; **CP**–Child's Preoccupation.

*of a terrorist attack).* CRT was specified by three indicators: The Child's General Fear Scale (CGFS), The Child's Everyday Fear Scale (CEFS) and Child's Preoccupation Scale (CPS). Also PRT was specified by three indicators: the parents' general anxiety scale (PAS), parents' control of child behavior (PCS), and parents' informative overloading (PILS). In this unrecursive model, the paths are directed to both sides: from PRT and FRT to CRT, and from CRT to PRT and FRT.

The unrecursive model indicated that CRT had a statistically significant effect on both PRT (standardized regression weight was .86, p = .000), and FRT (standardized regression weight was .64, p = .000). PRT and FRT did not have a statistically significant effect on CRT: standardized regression weights were .03, p = .842; and .02, p = .762.

Thus, results of the analysis of the structural equation models indicated that perceived reactions of parents and friends to terrorist attacks is not a mediator variable between PTE of the terrorist attack and the reactions of children. The results support the projection hypothesis that children project their reaction to terrorist attacks on their parents and friends and attribute to their parents and friends their fears and attitudes.

## DISCUSSION

*Relatively low level of fear and absence of pathological changes in behavior.* The prevalence rate and intensity of fear were found to be relatively low in our study. Pathological changes in children's behavior were not found (according to Achenbach's Child Behavioral Checklist).

Similar results were found in the research of reactions to long-term danger (war, daily terror) versus reaction to a sudden and isolated terrorist attack. A relatively low level of fear leads to a high level of coping and adaptation in conditions of long-term danger. War and prolonged terror do not always lead to mental and behavioral problems (Weisaeth, 1997). The study confirms that whereas only a small portion of the population suffers from mental breakdown or severe pathology, a greater proportion suffers from mild forms of stress, often of relatively brief duration (Zeidner, 1993). Also, a preliminary report based on a study of 2,422 school children (ages 7-17) in Kuwait during the Gulf War of 1990-1991 emphasized that 38% of the children reported having experienced fear for their lives (Weisaeth, 1997). These findings are consistent with observations of children in wars in many other places in the world, like Croatia, Cambodia, Central America and others.

Increased rates of alcohol abuse, smoking, stress, and PTSD were reported after each isolated sudden terrorist attack: Oklahoma City bombing (North et al., 1999; Smith et al., 1999); and after 1993 World Trade Center bombing (Koplewicz et al., 2002); after events of September 11, 2001 (Lerner, Gonzalez, Small & Fischhoff, 2003; Murphy, Wismar & Freeman, 2003; Schlenger et al., 2002; Schuster et al., 2001).

The object of our measuring was self-reported fear; however, it is very probable that social desirability influenced the results, an assumption supported by data indicating an attribution asymmetry effect found in a few studies (e.g., Shamai, 2002). In our study, children attributed more fears to their parents than to themselves and vice versa, parents attributed more fears to their children than to themselves.

*Differences of fear manifestation in various spheres of personality.* High internal consistency was found to exist between reactions to terror in various spheres of personality: emotional cognitive (CGFS), emotional-behavior (CEFS), behavioral (CPS) and cognitive (CWC). However, there were also significant differences between reactions in terms of their intensity and the factors determining the various reactions. Prevalence and intensity of general fear was higher than that of everyday fear. General fear was mainly determined by close emotional context (parent anxiety, friend anxiety). Everyday fear was mainly determined by parental control and situational factors related to a new terrorist attack. These differences remained, even when gender and age were controlled. Possible explanations follow.

1. Differences in the level of general and daily fears are by definition distinct types of fear: CGFS is reported as an overall cognitive apprehension about possible and probable danger; CEFS is reported as avoidance of specific, concrete forms of everyday activities.
2. These data correspond to the results obtained in the research of Muris and co-authors (2002), who used three different methods to assess these fears: Standard FSSC-R; Fear List Procedure (children were given a blank sheet of paper and asked to write down all stimuli and situations they feared); and the Calendar Procedure (children were given a weekly calendar on which they were requested to indicate retrospectively on which days they had been fearful of the five FSSC-R Danger and Death items). Results demonstrated that while these fears ranked high when using the standard FSSC-R procedure, they were considerably less common when using the Fear List Procedure and had a low probability of actual occurrence on a daily basis. In addition, fears were of short duration and low intensity (Muris et al., 2002). Results indicated that 50% of the children reported fear of "bombing attacks/being invaded" in FSSC-R (most common fear), whereas only 8% reported the same using the List Procedure and 2.9% using the Calendar Procedure. A possible explanation is that different methods measured various types of fear: FSSC-R measured general emotion-cognitive apprehension about possible danger, while the Fear

List Procedure and Calendar Procedure both measured the occurrence of actual manifestations of fear on a daily basis.

3. Influence of social desirability on results was higher in regard to fear of everyday activity (avoidance of everyday activity as a consequence of fear has connotation of "cowardice," "weakness") than general fear (acknowledgment, cognitive apprehension about real danger has connotation of wisdom, prudence, and caution, rather than of weakness).

*Children's self-reported fears and children's perception of their parents' reactions.* Children attribute to their parents a higher intensity and more prevalence of terror related fear than they do to themselves. The results of the analysis of the structural equation models support the projection hypothesis, in that they suggest that children project their reaction to terrorist attacks on their parents and friends and attribute to their parents and friends their own fears and attitudes.

These findings can be explained by the influence of social desirability. As mentioned, parents also attributed more fears to their children than to themselves (Shamai, 2002). An additional possible explanation might be the use of projection defense mechanism. What might be happening here is a cycle process of projecting identification, a concept which was developed by Melanie Klein in 1947. We refer to the model of Ogden (1986), in which parents and children are partners in the cycle of anxiety projected and planted in each other.

Shamai (2001) also explained the fact that parents attributed more fears to their children than to themselves by alluding to the projection mechanism. Parents unconsciously project their feeling onto the children simply by being busy with the children rather than self-engaged.

*A new terrorist attack has very little influence on children's fears.* A new terrorist attack does not produce significant additional fears in children. Place of residence, belonging to the community where the terrorist attack occurs, level of disruption, and time scope, in most cases, do not impact children's reactions.

A partial explanation of the findings may be attributed to the adaptive function of the defense mechanism. This may help the child to function in the short term. Anna Freud (1966) claimed that due to habit, the defenses become hardened; hence the child learns to filter the additional stimulations. Freud (1914), as well as Melanie Klein (1947), suggested that humans had both a drive for life and a drive for death, which are in constant struggle one with the other. When there are many situations that threaten life and introduce the certainty and fear of death, children hold on very strongly to their life drive in their inner world. Thus, they are able to overcome their fear of death.

An additional explanation relates to the influence of social desirability on the results. In a society like Israel, there is no place for expressions of fear related to threatening situations, because of heroic myths established and ingrained since the middle of the last century.

## CONCLUSION

As our findings have shown, currently children report reasonable levels of fear, a fact which enables them to adapt and adjust to daily life in conditions of prolonged terror. Nevertheless, there is a set of situations that prevents us from an optimistic assessment of the findings. First, fear of terror is habitual for many Israeli children. Second, reported fears of terror are significantly decreased by the influence of social desirability, heroic myths, mechanisms of defense, and children's projection of their fears onto their parents. Third, we do not know anything about profound internal consequences of living in conditions of daily terror on the psychology, world outlook, choice of strategies, and adaptive behavior of children in either the short or the long-term. Fourth, personal differences in the reactions of children to daily terror remain unstudied.

In future studies, we hope to research the links between reported fears of terror and the neuro-physiological state of children, their personal characteristics, and behavior strategies in different situations.

## REFERENCES

Achenbach, T.M. and Edellnock, C. (1987). *Manual for the youth self-report and profile*. University of Vermont, Department of Psychiatry, Burlington, VT.

Barenbaum, J., Ruchkin, V. and Schwab-Stone, M. (2004). The psychosocial aspects of children exposed to war: Practice and policy initiatives. *Journal of Child Psychology and Psychiatry*, 45(1), 41-62.

Bleich, A., Gelkopf, M. and Solomon, Z. (2003). Exposure to terrorism, stress-related mental health symptoms, and coping behavior among a nationally representative sample in Israel. *Journal of the American Medical Association*, 290, 612-620.

Desivilya, H.S., Gal, R. and Ayalon, O. (1996). Long-term effects of trauma in adolescence: Comparison between survivors of terrorist attack and control counterparts. *Anxiety, Stress and Coping*, 9: 135-150.

Freid, A. (1966). *The ego and the mechanisms of defense.* International Universities Press, New York.

Galea, S. and Resnick, H. (2005). Posttraumatic stress disorder in the general population after mass terrorist incidents: Considerations about the nature of exposure. *CNS Spectrums. International Journal of Neuropsychiatric Medicine,* 10(2), 107-115.

Gidron, V. (2002). Posttraumatic stress disorders after terrorist attacks: A review. *Journal of Nervous and Mental Disease,* 190(2): 118-121.

Jones, R., Ribbe, D. and Cunningham, P. (1994). Psychosocial correlates of fire disaster among children and adolescents. *Journal of Traumatic Stress,* 7(1): 117-122.

Joshi, P.T. and O'Donnell, D.A. (2003). Consequences of child exposure to war and terrorism. *Clinical Child and Family Psychology Review,* 6(4): 275-292.

Keinan, G., Sadeh, A. and Rosen, S. (2003). Attitudes and reactions to media coverage of Terrorist acts. *Journal of Community Psychology,* 31: 49-165.

Klein, M. (1959). *The psychoanalysis of children.* Hogarth Press, London.

Koplewicz, H.S., Vogel, J.M., Solanto, M.V., Morrissey, R.F., Alonso, C.M., Abikoff, H., Gallagher, R. and Novick, R.M. (2002). Child and parent response to the 1993 World Trade Center Bombing. *Journal of Traumatic Stress,* 15(1): 77-85.

Lerner, J., Gonzalez, R., Small, D. and Fischhoff, B. (2003). Effects of fear and anger on perceived risks of terrorism: A national field experiment. *Psychological-Science,* 14(2): 144-150.

McCathe, H. and Spence, S.H. (1991). What is the Revised Fear Survey Schedule for Children Measuring? *Behavior Research and Therapy,* 29: 495-502.

Muris, P., Merckelbach, H., Ollendick, T.H., King, N.J., Meestrs, C. and van Kessel, C. (2002). What is the Revised Fear Survey Schedule for Children Measuring? *Behavior Research and Therapy,* 40: 1317-1326.

Muris, P. and Ollendick, T. H. (2002). The assessment of contemporary fears in adolescents using a modified version of the Fear Survey Schedule for Children-Revised. *Journal of Anxiety Disorders,* 16(5): 567-584.

Muris, P., Meesters, C., Mayer, B., Bogie, N., Luijten, M., Geebelen,E., Bessems, J. and Smit, C. (2003). The Kola Fear Questionnaire: A standardized self-report scale for assessing fears and fearfulness in pre-school and primary school children. *Behavior Research and Therapy,* 41: 597-617.

Murphy, R., Wismar, K. and Freeman, K. (2003). Stress symptoms among African-American college students after the September 11, 2001 terrorist attacks. *Journal of Nervous and Mental Disease,* 191(2): 108-114.

North, C., Nixon S., Shariat, S., Mallonee, S., McMillen, J., Spitzanagel, E. and Smith, E. (1999). Psychiatric disorders among survivors of the Oklahoma City bombing. *Journal of the American Medical Association,* 282(8): 755-762.

Ogden, T.H. (1986). *The matrix of the mind: Object relations and the psychoanalytic dialogue.* Northvale, London.

Ollendick, T. H. (1983). Reliability and validity of the Fear Survey Schedule for Children-Revised (FSSC-R). *Behavior Research and Therapy,* 21: 685-692.

Ryan-Wenger, N. (2001). Impact of threat of war on children in military families. *American Journal of Orthopsychiatry,* 71(2): 236-244.

Schlenger, W. E., Caddell, J. M., Ebert, L., Jordan, B. K., Rourke, K. M., Wilson, D., Thalji, L., Dennis, J. M., Fairbank, J. A. and Kulka, R. A. (2002). Psychological reactions to terrorist attacks: Findings from the National Study of Americans' Reactions to September 11. *Journal of the American Medical Association*, 288(5): 581-588.

Schuster, M. A., Stein, B. D., Jaycox, L., Collins, R. L., Marshall, G.N., Elliott, M.N., Zhou, A.J., Kanouse, D.E., Morrison, J.L. and Berry, S.H. (2001). A national survey of stress reactions after the September 11, 2001, terrorist attacks. *New England Journal of Medicine*, 345(20): 1507-1512.

Shamai, M. (2002). Parents' perceptions of their children in a context of shared political uncertainty: The case of Jewish settlers in the West Bank before and after the Oslo peace agreement. *Child and Adolescence Social Work*, 19(1): 57-75.

Slone, M. (2000). Response to media coverage of terrorism. *Journal of Conflict Resolution*, 44(4): 508-522.

Smith, D., Christiansen, E., Vincent, R. and Hann, N. (1999). Population effects of the bombing of Oklahoma City. *Journal of the Oklahoma State Medical Association*, 92: 193-198.

Solomon, Z. and Lavi, T. (1999). Children in war: Soldiers against their will. In: Maercker, A., Schutzwohl, M. and Solomon, Z. (Eds.), *Posttraumatic stress disorder: A lifespan development perspective*. Hogrefe and Huber, Washington.

Terr, L.C. (1991). Childhood traumas: An outline and overview. *American Journal of Psychiatry*, 148, 10-20.

Tobin, J. (2000). Observations on the mental health of a civilian population living under long-term hostilities. *Psychiatric-Bulletin*, 24(2): 69-70.

Walter, G.D. (2002). Fear, belief, and terrorism. In: Shocov, S.P. (Ed.). *Advances in psychology research*, Vol. 10. Nova Science Publishers, Huntington, NY. pp. 45-67.

Weisaeth, L. (1997). War-related psychopathology in Kuwait: An assessment of war-related mental health problems. In: Fullerton, C.S. and Ursano, R.J. (Eds.) *Posttraumatic stress disorder: Acute and long-term responses to trauma and disaster*. American Psychiatric Press, Washington. pp. 91-121.

Ziender, M. (1993). Coping with disaster: The case of Israeli adolescents under threat of missile attack. *Journal of Youth and Adolescence*, 22(1): 89-108.

# Social Workers Confront Terrorist Victims:
# The Interventions and the Difficulties

Nelly Fraidlin, MA
Barbara Rabin, MA

**SUMMARY.** The article deals with unremitting stress experienced by social workers dealing with terror victims.

The article will describe the activity of social workers responsible for setting up a hospital information center. It will describe how they assist families searching for their loved ones and the process of identifying victims.

The process in which the uncertainty is treated, the anxiety is contained, bad news is conveyed and concrete solutions are provided, will be elaborated on.

Special emphasis will be placed on the multifaceted complimentary relationship between team members and between the provision of support, role exchange and the opportunity to share difficult experiences.

The team is expert in identifying both personal and collective signs of distress. This is of particular significance and importance in connection with compassion fatigue, survival guilt, anxiety, depression and on-going burnout, regarding themselves and their colleagues.

Nelly Fraidlin is Deputy Director of the Social Services Department, responsible for the Information Center, Sapir Medical Center, Meir Hospital, Kfar Saba, Israel (E- mail: nellyfr@clalit.org.il). Barbara Rabin is Director of the Social Services Department, Sapir Medical Center, Meir Hospital, Kfar Saba, Israel (E-mail: barbarara@clalit.org.il).

The authors would like to acknowledge the professional assistance provided by the Social Work Department of Mount Sinai Hospital. In addition, the authors would like to thank Professor Helen Rehr for her support and valuable input.

[Haworth co-indexing entry note]: "Social Workers Confront Terrorist Victims: The Interventions and the Difficulties." Fraidlin, Nelly, and Barbara Rabin. Co-published simultaneously in *Social Work in Health Care* (The Haworth Press, Inc.) Vol. 43, No. 2/3, 2006, pp. 115-130; and: *International Social Health Care Policy, Programs, and Studies* (ed: Gary Rosenberg, and Andrew Weissman) The Haworth Press, Inc., 2006, pp. 115-130. Single or multiple copies of this article are available for a fee from The Haworth Document Delivery Service [1-800-HAWORTH, 9:00 a.m. - 5:00 p.m. (EST). E-mail address: docdelivery@haworthpress.com].

Available online at http://swhc.haworthpress.com
© 2006 by The Haworth Press, Inc. All rights reserved.
doi:10.1300/J010v43n02_08

The article will propose organizational and clinical solutions, which could also be of service to other frameworks within the health system. *[Article copies available for a fee from The Haworth Document Delivery Service: 1-800-HAWORTH. E-mail address: <docdelivery@haworthpress.com> Website: <http:// www.HaworthPress.com>* © *2006 by The Haworth Press, Inc. All rights reserved.]*

**KEYWORDS.** Victims, information center, families, social workers

Health care workers, in order to prevent compassion fatigue and offer a state of the art service, usually build a sense of defense around them, enabling them to deal with their daily tasks. However at times of extreme stress, such as terror attacks, they themselves can be affected by the implications of these events and be susceptible to a variety of stress related, psychological symptoms (Hammond & Brooks, 2001). Fear, uncertainty and demoralization are feelings brought up by terrorism and this confronts social workers as well (Marshall & Suh, 2003). Saakvitne (2002) maintains that trauma experienced both by the social worker and his/her client exacerbates the social worker's difficulties.

In focus groups in Israel, both social work and nursing population groups have supported these feelings (Riba & Reches, 2002; Peled-Avram et al., 2004). Restoring a lost sense of personal security in order to resume professional performance, meeting family's tragedies and responding to it and disconnecting emotionally in order to promote the professional self, are all means of coping (Somer, 2004).

In a study on social workers following September 11 attacks, Boscarino et al. (2004) maintains that a supportive work environment is an important factor in preventing secondary trauma. Policy in stress management is highly recommended (Riba & Reches, 2002).

In Israel, state policy and hospital management have developed "Information Centers" providing a service to the public. The "Information Center" is the name given to the function fulfilled by social workers during the course of a terrorist attack or another multi casualty event, and it embraces several activities.

During the first hours following a terrorist attack, both the casualties and their families react out of shock, anxiety, panic and disorientation. This is a crisis situation whose very nature requires immediate, concrete and practical intervention. Being informed is the social worker's primary means to deal with a family member in crisis.

The "Information Center" operates out of several locations:

- The casualty ward (where the victims are taken in);
- The Information Center headquarters;
- The telephone response center;
- The site where families are received and the pictures of the uniden-tifiable victims are shown;
- The site where victims suffering from stress are taken care of.

Each site will be described according to three parameters:

- The main task of the social worker in the site.
- The professional role.
- The difficulties and dilemmas in the site.

This paper deals with social workers and their task difficulties and di-lemmas at times of terrorist attacks. It offers a conceptual model of op-erating at this critical time.

## *CASUALTY RECEPTION SITE (THE E.R.)*

This is the emergency ward where terror victims are taken in and which provides initial medical treatment designed to stabilize their con-dition.

*The principal tasks* for the social worker at this location are:

The provision of assistance in establishing contact between the victim and their families, provision of assistance in identifying victims and providing a response to the victim's special needs.

### *The Role*

*Assistance in Establishing Contact Between the Victims and Their Families*

In the case of the lightly injured, the social worker will encourage the victims to contact their families so, that these are able to hear their voices with the least possible delay, and learn, firsthand, about their condition. The casualties must be assisted in making this first contact, and in gaining coherence and control of the situation, while taking into consideration the emotional state of the person on the other end of the line. For this reason it is important that the emergency ward social worker support them.

It is the social worker's responsibility, to cross-check data received from staff at the family reception site, and to inform the latter (when the condition of the casualties permit) when families can be reunited, since it is important for both parties to be prepared for the meeting.

It frequently happens that more than one member of a single family is injured, and it is then the emergency ward social worker's responsibility to locate the related injured parties, in the different emergency wards, and to gently support the reunion.

Because these are difficult and sensitive situations, we try to "attach" a support worker to each family so that the latter will have a single person to turn to, for assistance and information.

Another role taken by the social worker, at this site, is to accompany patients to medical treatment, or to the stress center.

### Assistance in Identifying Victims

One of the principal functions of the social worker at the emergency ward, is to assist in the identification of casualties–such casualties from whom it is not possible to extract information, because they are in shock, confused, unconscious or severely injured.

The emergency ward social workers employ various and creative means of identifying the victims: they search for identifying documents, special items such as jewelry, special clothing and body marks, such as tattoos, piercing, birth marks, etc. (and then inform the "family site," about those signs, in order to help the searching families identify their loved ones).

### Responding to the Victim's Special Needs

In order to ease their period of staying in the emergency room, it is the social worker's responsibility, to provide a response to the victim's special personal problems and needs; issues which relate to their life beyond the confines of the hospital. The terrorist act which was perpetrated during the routine of a regular day's activity, filled with daily tasks, interrupt the course of normal activity, leaving unresolved matters at home, which must be taken care of: children at kindergarten, an elderly person who needs to be cared for, or a family member who needs, for example, to receive his daily insulin injection.

These are only a few examples of how the routine of daily life is suddenly violated, and how further stress is brought to bear on the victims, who are now unable to handle the normal daily tasks for which they alone are responsible.

## Difficulties and Dilemmas

The principal difficulties faced by the social worker at the site are several.

Her exposure to terrible scenes–blood, body parts, and scraps of clothing–is all totally ineradicable from her memory. It is extremely difficult to confront the shocked and confused victims. On the other hand, each victim must be given in-depth and personal attention, together with a large number of other victims.

A further difficulty is observing the emotional meetings between the victims and their families. This experience raises a storm of feelings in the support worker–confusion, disorientation, dissociation are common (Marmar et al., 1996).

The media is also another obstacle in this site, because there is much interest to cover the event authentically, and first hand. The reporters insist on interviewing the wounded, and photographing them, even though they are still in a state of shock.

# INFORMATION CENTER HEADQUARTERS

## Central Task

The principal function of the social worker at this site is data processing–ensuring that she/he is provided with a full list of both the identified and unidentified casualties, from both our own and from other hospitals (those hospitals which also admitted, simultaneously, casualties during the course of the event). This function is essential ensuring that full information on casualties admitted to the hospital is available for the families, and enabling crosschecking of data of unidentified casualties with families.

## The Role

The headquarters also maintain contact with external bodies to which it reports, on the casualties admitted to the hospital, such as police, army, municipality, government offices, etc.

Contact with other hospitals is also important, since they, too, need to use our lists and descriptions of unidentified casualties to assist families seeking their loved ones among those admitted to our hospital, and to help us, identifying casualties who were admitted there.

We inform the N.I.I. (National Insurance Institute) about the list of the casualties, the day after the event, in order to maintain a continuation of treatment, psychologically, socially, and financially.

### Difficulties and Dilemmas

The difficulties at this site are several.

The social worker's principal problem is associated with its seclusion. For logistical reasons and because of the sensitivity of the information, the headquarter is located at a considerable distance from the casualty wards and the family reception sites. The social worker confronts loneliness, uncertainty and helplessness (Fox, 2003; Myers & Wee, 2002) at the site, dealing with names only without seeing the people or their families.

At this site the social workers are under intense pressure to supply updated lists, to provide information to internal and external bodies. The social worker copes with a large amount of data, and many logistical problems. Since the information is sensitive, she/he has to decide what information to pass to whom. A further source of stress is the fear that the social worker will discover a familiar name on the lists.

## THE TELEPHONE SITE

### Central Task

This is the location from where telephone information is provided to families, by means of an emergency telephone number announced in the media.

The central task of this site is to provide immediate response to callers and to respond to the flood of telephone calls. This is usually the first site that is opened up and the last to be closed.

### The Role

There are few functions at this site:

- There is a need to immediate organization of emergency telephone lines and computers.

- Providing an adequate response even when there is only vague and ambiguous information.
- The social worker has to address the callers' emotional state, in an adequate and empathetic manner.
- Supplying the caller with other useful phone numbers for their continued search for more information.

## Difficulties and Dilemmas

In spite of the fact that on the face of it, the social worker at the telephone site is not required to face the sights, sounds and smells, nevertheless questions asked over the telephone–especially by people who were witness to the event (and who are still shocked and confused, the sights still pursuing them)–are frequently spine chilling and demand detachment, resourcefulness and self-control (Marmar et al., 1996).

It must be understood that it is frequently necessary to provide an appropriate, calming, and sympathetic response, while taking into account the agitated state of the caller, even though information is still unavailable and the facts still unclear. It is of course not easy to choose an ideal manner in which to divulge difficult and sensitive information, while unable to actually see the person on the other end of the line.

As a policy, the social workers are not allowed to give any information about the casualties. They inform the family that their loved one was admitted to our hospital. Here the social workers also face another difficulty–they must provide minimum information even though they may be aware of additional details, such as the condition of the casualty. Needless to say, they are totally prohibited from transmitting any details on fatalities, even when their identity is known. All these require a high level of self-control, and restraint.

## FAMILY RECEPTION SITE

### The Central Task

The social worker's principal task at this site is the furnishing of information to the families while providing them with help and support in seeking their relatives.

### The Role

The social worker is required to maintain an updated list of the casualties including those who were evacuated to other hospitals. She/he must locate families, whose response to a situation of uncertainty is more disturbed. She/he must support them and also identify and respond to their special needs.

As soon as it becomes clear, that a member of a waiting family is among the hospitalized casualties, the family must be informed gently and carefully. They must be made prepared for the meeting and be accompanied to the ward.

It is frequently necessary to provide concrete assistance such as ensuring that the family is accompanied to another hospital, or to accompany them to "Abu Kabir," that is the pathological institute. It is the place where the dead bodies are located; bodies of those who were killed on the spot, and did not reach a hospital.

An especially difficult moment is that when the social worker realizes that she/he must refer the family to Abu-Kabir. The association means death, and referring the family there is an awful task, something that every family lives in fear of hearing, and every social worker of having to notify.

### Difficulties and Dilemmas

The social worker's principal difficulty at this site are the tragedies they are forced to observe–witnessing some of the most unbearable moments ever to be experienced by the families. One of the most painful encounters is with those families who have not found the names of their loved ones among the lists, but who nevertheless strongly suspect that they were at the site of the attack. It is hard to face families over a lengthy period of time, who expect to be provided with information.

This is the site where the most difficult tidings are delivered: of severe injury and of death. The announcement of the news to the family is a traumatic experience for the social worker, too. The essence of emotional distress experienced by the social worker is knowing that they have to contain grief, tragedy, threat and anxiety of the family members (Peled Avram et al., 2004).

Another of the difficulties is "over-identification" with the families, especially those families "similar" to the social worker's background.

For every casualty, several relatives may visit the site to conduct a search and a larger circle of family and friends will come along to support them. The social workers at the site must also, therefore, simultaneously handle a large number of people requiring information and support.

The family's tragedy, its pain and loss, and severe shock are also traumatic experiences for those who deliver the news and for anyone else around. The repeated recurrence of such events produces unremitting stress among social workers.

Teenagers are often involved, and their friends will want to spend time with them at the hospital. A flood of teenagers requires special care, and special attention must be given to containment of their anxiety.

This site places special emphasis on contact with community social workers: in locating relatives who have not reached the hospital, and assistance in getting there, in notifying relatives at home, in accompanying relatives who might otherwise continue the search alone at other hospitals and, of course, accompanying them to Abu Kabir. We also employ the assistance of community workers in providing solutions to problems at home (such as for dependents of the casualty who require appropriate care) or needs identified at the hospital which need to be taken care of, within the community–such as injured children or infants who, to further intensify the tragedy, have lost their parents, and who require community support, both formal and informal.

## THE "SITE OF THE UNIDENTIFIED VICTIMS" (WHERE THE IDENTIFICATION TAKES PLACE)

### Central Task

Providing help identifying the unidentified victims by combining information from the emergency room, with information provided by the families.

This is a very traumatic place as usually those who are identified are either dead or badly wounded.

### The Role

The main roles include gathering information from the E.R. about particular signs of recognition, and cross checking them with the families and accompanying the families to the identification room, where photographs of the unidentified are presented, and then accompanying the family to the site where their loved one is located, it might be the surgical ward, or pathology.

## Difficulties and Dilemmas

Facing the uncertainty with which the families have to deal is a hard task, as well as the difficulty in accompanying the families to see the photographs and to meet their love ones, live or dead.

It is even harder to conceal information on deaths until full identification has been made, to accompany the family, which is anxiously attempting to identify personal items. The expectation that this "John Doe" is theirs, the disappointment when some other family makes a positive identification–are all very demanding, causing the social worker both emotional and physical exhaustion.

## STRESS VICTIMS SITE

### Central Task

The principal task at this site is to attempt to assess the emotional state of the casualties, to assist them in getting through the traumatic experience and to oversee their monitored release from hospital, while ensuring that they receive uninterrupted treatment.

In this area, psychiatrists of the hospital conduct together with social workers, a unique model of treatment whereby every casualty, admitted to the hospital as the result of a terrorist attack, will attend the stress victim's site, where his/her discharge will be formalized.

### The Role

Here conversations are held with the casualties in an attempt to get them to speak, both, one-on-one and in groups, and here they are given an opportunity to de-brief and ventilate. Here casualties with severe and extreme reactions are identified. Subsequently the casualty will be released but not before it is ascertained where he/she intends to go, with whom and how. Families of the stress victims are managed on a psycho-educational level within a group setting. This takes place optimally at the same time when their loved ones are being assessed and treated by the psychiatrists.

The community representatives from the welfare agencies in the area assist the hospital workers, in order to help discharge these victims in the best possible way.

Proper release of patients is no less important than their reception. They will be given relevant addresses, to which they may turn for further professional assistance, should they require it.

## Difficulties and Dilemmas

There are several difficulties in this site, such as working with other professionals, and staying long hours, until every victim is discharged properly. But the main difficulty is in confronting the descriptions and reconstructions of the terrible events experienced by the casualties. In a certain respect, the social worker experiences a form of "secondary trauma," as they are repeatedly exposed to the awful events. Although they were not physically at the site of the event, it is reconstructed for them, in all its force, and it is "almost" as if they were there.

This repeated experience can awaken emotional reactions in the social worker, often similar to those experienced by the victims who were actually present. This experience is influenced both by the background and culture of the worker him/herself, as well as the client. Our center has given special attention to this issue. We have staff members from different nationalities who both speak the language and understand various cultures. This allows us to be sensitive and treat a variety of responses such as: the quiet Ethiopian, who needed help to verbalize and express his feelings; the North African mother, whose demonstrative reaction could be adequately contained; the Russian soldier, who internalized his grief; and the religious family, whose faith helped them through.

Both staff members and terror victims might include Jews and Arabs. This situation magnifies the ambivalent feelings existing in the community.

Israel is a melting pot for different nationalities and new immigrants. This population is at particular risk because they lack support systems and may not be adequately oriented to the new country. Cross-cultured reactivation of trauma has a significant clinical impact (Kinzie et al., 2002).

## CONCLUSION

The recurring confrontation of hospital social workers with terror victims is a harrowing experience.

Such repeated incidents are capable of producing severe reactions among social workers, to a certain extent, similar to those experienced by the casualties themselves. Social workers can experience sorrow and anger, which needs to be identified before offering assistance to others (Ming-sum & Fernando, 2003).

It must be understood that a multiple casualty event is characterized by indescribable stress, both concrete stress in the need to simultaneously handle a large number of people in pain, shock and confusion, and emotional stress in face of the uncertainty and anxiety experienced by the families.

In spite of the parallel processes, which confront the social worker in his/her work with the casualties and their families, they must maintain maximum control of the situation, and preserve their composure while performing their work to the highest standard; they must assess and diagnose the condition of the people they confront, handle situations of uncertainty, contain anxieties, support people in their pain, deliver terrible news with maximum sensitivity, while at the same time providing concrete solutions to a multitude of needs. Repeated exposure to these situations are capable of creating emotional reactions among the social workers, characteristic of exposure to "secondary trauma": trauma experienced not by someone who directly experienced the event but rather by indirect exposure (Hodgkinson & Shepherd, 1994).

According to Terr (1989), indirect exposure to a traumatic event occurs when someone happens to see the psychiatric symptoms, defenses and emotional stress that accompany someone else's psychiatric trauma.

And indeed, social workers at the various sites report depression and exhaustion. Bleich and Kutz (2002) emphasize the importance of taking care of the carers. In the period immediately after an incident, they may suffer from sleep problems and lack of appetite. Any terrorist attack, even if it takes place a long way from the home hospital, reawakens these same reactions. The literature speaks of "compassion fatigue" and "survival guilt" experienced by those who, time after time are required to take care of the casualties (Figley, 1995). This phenomenon is expressed by confusion, helplessness, isolation from support systems and psychosomatic symptoms (Lahad & Ayalon, 1994).

Harris (1995) claims that empathy is the key factor that causes intrusion to the therapist's reactions. The fact that the casualties might be similar to the health professional worker on many parameters places him at high risk.

According to Lahad and Aayalon (1994), and Kfir (1990), the main causes of the difficulties of the workers are the conditions of the intervention: intensive, immediate, and unlimited in time.

Many times the team members live geographically close to the area and this make them a "near miss" and cause a strong identification, which interferes with their ability to be detached from the event.

## RECOMMENDATIONS

The health setting dealing with the mass casualty should develop an infrastructure that enables its workers to cope more effectively with the impact of the disaster. We suggest three parameters: behavioral, cognitive, and emotional that should be regarded.

### *The Behavioral Domain*

There are several ways that from an operational point of view the social work team can deal with the after effects of the multi-causality event. Social workers have developed several tools designed to ease the suffering even though these programs have been under debate especially over the past ten years. In particular, debriefing has been researched and found that its efficacy is controversial (Van Emmerik et al., 2002; Deahl, 2000; Bisson, 2003). It is important to examine time and duration of the meeting, population characteristics, group leaders and their ability, content and process of the group and outcome measures before making a final decision (Hammond & Brooks, 2002; Dekel et al., 2004). It offers a sense of togetherness with those who have experienced a similar situation and reduces the feeling of loneliness. It transmits the event to something that can be controlled and understood (Peled Avram et al., 2004).

From our experience, immediately after the event, before the staff goes home, it is important for all those involved, in a group session to sit and share their experiences and ventilate. This gives a sense of belonging, a place to express their own sorrow and offers a feeling of togetherness (Mitchell & Bary, 1990; Mitchell & Dyregrov, 1993; Van Emmerik et al., 2002; Kaplan et al., 2001).

The next day, as practised in our setting, once again the staff should meet to discuss in a more organized way, their coping mechanisms. This is also the time to learn how the event was handled on a technical level and to learn from this process (Lahad & Ayalon, 1994).

## *The Cognitive Domain*

Although the literature is skeptical concerning trauma training and ongoing formal education (Dekel et al., 2004), the staff should be exposed to a workshop dealing specifically with vicarious traumatization. In the same way that trauma disrupts the cognitive schema of the victim, the concept of vicarious traumatization suggests that exposure to a client's trauma can, over time, lead to disruption in the clinician's cognitive schemas (McCann & Pearlman, 1990; Pearlman & Saakvitne in Cunningham, 2003; Pearlman & Maclan, 1995). This workshop should be adapted to and built together with each team in the specific hospital. Each unit has its idiosyncratic approach and limitations and this needs to be taken into account.

Social workers who are identified as high risk for extreme reactions should be rotated among the various sites. Workers are different in their ability to cope with disaster and some of their functions need to be limited in order to reduce vicarious traumatization (Palm et al., 2004; Figley, 1995; McCann & Pearlman, 1990). Pearlman and Saakvitne (1995) provide an interactive approach to understanding the effect of trauma work on clinicians. It involves the interaction of the clinician's personal characteristics, life circumstances and personal history of trauma, along with the material presented by the client (in Cunningham, 2003).

Organizations need to recognize that training in trauma work can be a preventative measure for compassion fatigue as it conveys the message that vicarious traumatization is an expected reaction (Schauben & Frazier, 1995; Munroe in Cunningham, 2003; Ruzek, 2002; Palm et al., 2004).

## *The Emotional Domain*

An emphasis on strengths of the worker, including a sense of professional and self competence, being objective, resolving personal traumas, clear goals and professional, collegial support, should be encouraged (Bell, 2003).

There is no doubt that these events, which exhort an emotional price, constitute a very special risk for those who are exposed to them, time and time again in the course of their work. Workers should be encouraged to use their personal and familial resources to cope with the pressures of dealing with these events. Most important is sharing ones experiences with others and finding meaning in ones purpose in life (Palm et al., 2004).

It is important to rescue the rescuer.

# REFERENCES

Bell, H. (2003). Strengths and Secondary Trauma in Family Violence. *Social Work*, 48 (4), 513-522.

Bisson, J.I. (2003). Single-Session Early Psychological Interventions Following Traumatic Events. *Clinical Psychology Review*, 23 (3): 481-99.

Bleich, A. & Kutz, I. (2002). Chemical and Biological Terrorism: Psychological Aspects, a Guideline for Psychiatric Preparedness. *Harefuah*, 141 spec No: 111-7, 118 (Article in Hebrew).

Boscarino, J.A., Figley, C.R. & Adams, R.E. (2004). Compassion Fatigue Following the September 11 Terrorist Attacks: A Study of Secondary Trauma among New York City Social Workers. *International Journal of Emergency Mental Health*, 6 (2): 57-66.

Cunningham, M. (2003). Impact of Trauma Work on Social Work Clinicians: Empirical Findings. *Social Work*, 48 (4), 513-522.

Deahl, M. (2000). Psychological Debriefing: Controversy and Challenge. *Australian and New Zealand Journal of Psychiatry*, 34 (6): 929-39.

Dekel, R., Ginzburg, K. & Hentman, S. (2004). In the Front Line: Hospital Social Workers Confront Ongoing Terrorism. *Society and Welfare*, 24 (2), 163-180.

Figley, C.R. (1995). Compassion Fatigue as Secondary Traumatic Stress Disorder: An Overview. In C.R. Figley (Ed.), *Compassion Fatigue: Coping with Secondary Traumatic Disorder in Those who Treat the Traumatized* (pp. 1-20). New York: Brunner/ Mazel.

Fox, R. (2003). Traumaphobia: Confronting Personal and Professional Anxiety. *Psychoanalytic Social Work*, 10, 43-55.

Hammond J. & Brooks J. (2001). The World Trade Center Attack: Helping the Helpers: The Role of Critical Incident Stress Management. *Critical Care*, 5: 315-317.

Harris, C.J. (1995). Sensory Based Therapy for Crisis Counselors. In Figley, C.H. (Ed.). *Compassion Fatigue*. New York: Brunner/Mazel.

Hodgkinson, P.E. & Shepherd, M.A. (1994). The Impact of Disaster Support Work. *Journal of Trauma Stress*, 7 (4): 587-600.

Kaplan, Z., Iancu, I. & Bodner, E. (2001). A View of Psychological Debriefing after Extreme Stress. *Psychiatric Service*, 52 (6), 824-7.

Kfir, N. (1990). *Like Circles in the Water*. Tel-Aviv, Am Oved.

Kinzie, J.D., Boehnlein, J.K., Riley, C. & Sparr, L. (2002). The Effects of September 11 on Traumatized Refugees Reactive of Postraumatic Stress Disorder. *Journal of Nervous Mental Disorders*, July 190 (7): 437-41.

Lahad, M. & Ayalon, E. (1994*). About Life and Death*. Haifa, Nord Press.

Marmar, C.R., Weiss, D.S., Metzler, T. & Delucchi, K. (1996). Characteristics of Emergency Services Personnel Related to Peritraumatic Dissociation During Critical Incident Exposure. *The American Journal of Psychiatry*, 153, 94-102.

Marshall R.D. & Suh E.J. (2003). Contextualizing Trauma: Using Evidence-Based Treatments in Multicultural Community after 9/11. *Psychiatric Quarterly*, Winter 74 (4): 401-20.

McCann, L. & Pearlman, L.A. (1990). Vicarious Traumatization: A Framework for Understanding the Psychological Effects of Working with Victims. *Journal of Traumatic Stress*, 3, 131-149.

Ming-sum, T. & Fernando, C.H. (2003). Dealing with Terrorism: What Social Workers Should and Can Do. *Social Work*, 48 (4), 556-557.

Mitchell, J. & Bary, G. (1990). *Emergency Services Stress*. Englewood Clift. NJ: Prentice Hall.

Mitchell, J. & Dyregrov, A. (1993). Traumatic Stress in Disaster Workers and Emergency Personnel. In Wilson J. & Raphael B. (Eds) *The International Handbook of Traumatic Stress Sydrome*. New York: Plenum Press. 905-914.

Myers, D. G., & Wee, D.F. (2002). Strategies for Managing Disaster Mental Health Worker Stress. In C.R. Figley (Ed.), *Treating Compassion Fatigue* (pp. 181-211). New York: Brunner/ Routledge.

Palm, K.M., Polusny, M.A. & Follette, V.M. (2004). Vicarious Traumatization: Potential Hazards and Interventions for Disaster and Trauma Workers. *Prehospital and Disaster Medicine*, 19 (1), 73-78.

Pearlman, L.A., & Maclan, P.S. (1995). Vicarious Traumatization: An Empirical Study of the Effects of Trauma Work on Trauma Therapists. *Professional Psychology: Research and Practice*, 26, 558-565.

Pearlman, L.A. & Saakvitne, K. (1995). *Trauma and the Therapist: Contertransference and Vicarious Traumatization in Psychotherapy with Incest Survivors*. New York: W.W. Norton.

Peled-Avram, M., Ben Yitzhak, Y., Gagin, R., Zomer, E. & Buchbinder, E. (2004). Responses and Emotional Needs of Social Workers in the Face of Terrorist attacks with Multiple Casualities. *Society & Welfare*, 24 (2).

Riba, S. & Reches, H. (2002). When Terror is Routine: How Israeli Nurses Cope with Multi-Casuality Terror. *Online Journal of Issues in Nursing*, 7 (3).

Ruzek, J.I. (2002). Providing "Brief Education and Support" for Emergency Response Workers: An Alternative to Debriefing. *Military Medicine*, 167 (9 suppl): 73-5.

Saakvitne, K.W. (2002) Shared Trauma: The Therapist's Increased Vulnerability. *Psychoanalytic Dialogues*, 12, 443-449.

Schauben, L.J. & Frazier, P. (1995). Vicarious trauma: The Effects on Female Counselors of Working with Sexual Violence Survivors. *Psychology of Women Quarterly*, 19: 49-64.

Somer, E., Buchbinder, E, Peled-Avram, M. & Ben-Yizhack, Y. (2004) The Stress and Coping of Israeli Emergency Room Social Workers Following Terrorist Attacks. *Qualitative Health Research*, 14 (8): 1077-93.

Terr, L. (1989). Family Anxiety after Traumatic Events. *Journal of Clinical Psychiatric*, 50 (suppl.): 15-19.

Van Emmerik, A.A., Kamphuis, J.H., Hulsbosh, A.M. & Emmelkamp, P.M. (2002). Single Session Debriefing after Psychological Trauma: A Meta-Analysis. *Lancet*, Sep. 7, 360 (9335): 741-2.

# Learning from Each Other:
# The Social Work Role
# as an Integrated Part
# of the Hospital Disaster Response

Rosalie Pockett, PhD, MAASWAcc

**SUMMARY.** Australian social workers in health care have become important members of hospital disaster response teams. The development of the role and its integration into the mainstream disaster response has progressed over the last two decades. Recent international events have given affirmation to the importance of this role.

The development of national and state based disaster management plans in Australia began in the mid 1970s. Recognition of the need for experienced, skilled workers to provide emotional support, practical assistance and grief and bereavement counselling has resulted in the inclusion of social workers in several key parts of the disaster management response including the specialised area of disaster victim identification.

Rosalie Pockett is Lecturer, Social Work and Policy Studies, Faculty of Education and Social Work, The University of Sydney, NSW 2006, Australia (E-mail: rpockett@usyd.edu.au). The author is a scholar of the Mt. Sinai Leadership Enhancement Program (1993-4) and had study visits to Mt. Sinai in 1996 and 2001.

This paper was presented at the Doris Siegel Memorial Colloquium, Mt. Sinai Medical Center, NY, May 19th-20th, 2004.

This article is dedicated to the memory of Alison McMichael who died in Adelaide, South Australia in late 2004 after a long illness.

[Haworth co-indexing entry note]: "Learning from Each Other: The Social Work Role as an Integrated Part of the Hospital Disaster Response." Pockett, Rosalie. Co-published simultaneously in *Social Work in Health Care* (The Haworth Press, Inc.) Vol. 43, No. 2/3, 2006, pp. 131-149; and: *International Social Health Care Policy, Programs, and Studies* (ed: Gary Rosenberg, and Andrew Weissman) The Haworth Press, Inc., 2006, pp. 131-149. Single or multiple copies of this article are available for a fee from The Haworth Document Delivery Service [1-800-HAWORTH, 9:00 a.m. - 5:00 p.m. (EST). E-mail address: docdelivery@haworthpress.com].

Available online at http://swhc.haworthpress.com
© 2006 by The Haworth Press, Inc. All rights reserved.
doi:10.1300/J010v43n02_09

Following the Bali Bombing in October 2002, social workers worked with the police missing persons unit to provide support to families and facilitate the collection of ante mortem information.

The process by which new services come about can be intricate and complex. In the field of health social work, the contribution of international programs such as the Mt. Sinai Leadership Enhancement Program cannot be underestimated. As the Social Work Director of Westmead Hospital, one of the largest hospital social work departments in the country, participating in this program provided opportunities to share professional experience with international colleagues, many of whom are experts in their field.

The social work role in disaster response has become internationally recognised and is an example of how collaboration and shared information and learning can result in a profession working together to support key principles and values of practice for the benefit of those in need. *[Article copies available for a fee from The Haworth Document Delivery Service: 1-800-HAWORTH. E-mail address: <docdelivery@haworthpress.com> Website: <http://www.HaworthPress.com> © 2006 by The Haworth Press, Inc. All rights reserved.]*

**KEYWORDS.** Social work, disaster management, disaster victim identification, leadership enhancement program

## INTRODUCTION

Australian social workers in health care have become important members of hospital disaster response teams with a significant role in the immediate psycho-social care of disaster affected persons. The development of the role has occurred over the last two decades and recent international events have affirmed the significant contribution the role makes to a co-ordinated disaster response.

The Social Work Department at Westmead Hospital Sydney has developed a functional and tested plan drawing from international and national experience and the shared learning among the Alumni of the Mt. Sinai Leadership Program (Irrizarry, Gameau, and Walter 1993; Rehr and Epstein, 1993). The author was a scholar of the Program in 1993-4 with Australian social worker, Alison McMichael, and Israeli social worker, Margalit Drory.

## The Australian Experience of Disasters

The Australian experience of disasters has been a mixture of natural disasters, such as brush fires, floods, and cyclones, and catastrophic human events such as road and rail accidents that have resulted in large numbers of fatalities, serious injuries and property destruction.

In the 1970s two major disasters occurred. In December 1974 Cyclone Tracey hit the city of Darwin in the Northern Territory. Sixty-five people died, six hundred and fifty were injured and most of the forty-five thousand residents were evacuated. Much was learned from this event and the beginning stages of a national disaster response organisation emerged. Three years later, in 1977, at Granville Sydney, a commuter train crash challenged the coping capacity of the local hospitals to manage large numbers of casualties. Eighty-three passengers died and two hundred and thirteen were injured. From these two tragedies, national and state based disaster management plans were developed (Lennox, 1996; Hicks, 1998; Hodge, 2000; Lee and Collings, 2000).

These early disaster plans focused on immediate response and rescue. As other smaller scale incidents occurred, the plans began to include other aspects of disaster response including the care of 'non-injured' disaster affected persons, and the recovery of both victims and emergency services' personnel (Disaster Management Australia, 1999).

## LITERATURE REVIEW

Social workers have had key roles in responses to natural disasters (Sherraden and Fox, 1993; Beck and Franke, 1996). The skills used in these situations have been identified as advocacy, liaison with government and non-government agencies, community development and an understanding of the social needs of individuals and families who have experienced social dislocation. The goals of intervention have been focused on community recovery and restoration.

In a study by Steinglass and Gerrity (1990), cited in Beck and Franke (1996), between fifteen and twenty percent of persons studied after natural disasters were reported to have symptoms of post traumatic stress disorder (PTSD). The literature on trauma associated with disasters has been developing over the last two decades with Beck and Franke (1996) acknowledging that 'the entire body of empirical literature on trauma associated with disasters comes from the fields of Social Work and Psychology.'

The impact of disasters on communities and individuals has been further discussed in relation to human initiated disasters where the event is intentional (Jacobs and Kulkarni, 1999; O'Neill, 2001; Novick, 2003). In addition to the destruction of resources and property, and large scale loss of life, the dimension of fear is also present. Accompanying this is a deep sense of vulnerability and the loss of a sense of personal safety in the community. When responding to these types of events, social workers draw on their skills in crisis intervention providing emotional support and practical assistance to meet the immediate needs of disaster affected persons (Lindmann, 1944; Groner, 1978; Fein and Knautt, 1986; Truswell, Blyth, Kendall, and Shipway, 1988; Hepworth and Larson, 1996; Reyes Gilbert and Elhadi, 2004; Van Ommeren, Saxena, and Saraceno, 2005).

Drawing on the Israeli experience, Yanay and Benjamin (2005) comment that social workers 'deal with the social outcomes of disaster' and provide services to injured victims, their families and the survivors of those missing or killed. These services are provided within two interrelated frameworks. The first is the organizational framework and role of the leading agency assuming responsibility for relief operations and secondly the professional framework and formal and informal processes that the relief operation entails. The organizational framework is provided by the government and non-government agencies that come together in a planned and coordinated response. The literature reflects differences and similarities between countries in how these frameworks have been developed. These can best be viewed at the websites of such organizations as the American Red Cross, the Federal Emergency Management Agency (FEMA, US) and Emergency Management Australia.

The professional framework is provided by the practice skills and knowledge base that social workers bring to the disaster situation. The experience and skills of social workers in emergency rooms and intensive care units have been identified as being most relevant and applicable to the immediate response (Newburn, 1993; Ben Shahar, 1993; Boes, 1997; Somer, Buchbinder, Peled-Avram, and Ben-Yizhack, 2004). Key social work roles include providing information, practical support such as housing and financial assistance, and a range of therapeutic interventions such as validation, facilitation, and narration/story telling by victims, that contribute to the restoration of self-efficacy in the disaster victim.

Much of the contemporary Australian mental health literature recognizes the importance of immediate 'psychological first-aid' for disaster affected persons. This intervention is defined as follows: psychological first aid involves approaching and offering support to people involved in the incident, with a focus on the establishment of safety, the provision of practical help in meeting basic human needs and physical care, for example, food, shelter, and contact with loved ones. Supportive counselling is also provided. Supportive counselling is the provision of information and emotional support by a trained counsellor in order to support a person through a crisis or period of distress, and to refer for further assessment and management if necessary (NSW Health Plan, 2001).

A fundamental feature of effective intervention by social workers is the controlled 'use of self' that Yanay and Benjamin have identified; 'self-restraint, control and awareness are basic' to this intervention. The deployment of social workers to an emergency or disaster response must take into account the personal impact that events may have on the workers themselves as members of the community. Ensuring their own loved ones are safe prior to deployment is a priority of the Israeli response plan (Yanay & Benjamin, 2005). In a study investigating the stress and coping of Israeli Emergency Room social workers following terrorist attacks, Somer, Buchbiner, Peled-Avram and Ben-Yizhack (2004) held four focus groups with thirty-eight hospital social workers. Three themes emerged; restoring a lost sense of personal security as a necessary stepping-stone toward resuming professional performance; meeting the families' pain and responding to it; and disconnecting emotionally in the service of the professional self. The qualitative study demonstrated the personal impact of the work on the social workers. The results of this study support the findings of a study by Boscarino, Figley and Adams (2004) that secondary trauma was negatively associated with having a supportive work environment.

The Yanay and Benjamin study acknowledged that 'despite training, preparation and exposure to emergency situations some social workers were better equipped to handle the demanding situation than others.' The study recommended that only informed and consenting professionals who are at low risk of experiencing vicarious trauma should be asked to participate in this high risk work. Rubinstein (2004) also identified a number of personal qualities that social workers must have including a capacity to deal with uncertainty and a capacity to work in interdisciplinary and inter-cultural teams. Disaster victims and health professionals, who care for them, will reflect the heterogeneous mix of cultures and beliefs in the community in which the event occurred.

Another role for social workers is emerging within the context of the forensic medicine response to mass casualty events. Newhill and Sites (2000) discuss the role in a case study of an airline disaster in Pittsburgh in 1994 where the author was assigned as a social worker to the city morgue. The case study discussed the tasks undertaken by the social workers:

> The skills that social workers bring to the interdisciplinary disaster intervention team are based upon social work's historic practice in crisis situations (mostly with individuals and families) and are transferable to other settings. . . . As others have noted, social workers are exceptionally well prepared for disaster intervention because of their person-in-situation orientation (Baker and Zakour, 1996), familiarity with crisis theory, skill in working with people from a strengths perspective, and, perhaps especially because of their experience and comfort in approaching persons in the field. (p. 99)

The emergence of a social work specialization in disaster response has been recognized (Newhill and Sites 2000) along with the need for the inclusion of disaster training in the social work teaching curricula (Dodds and Neuring, 1996; Novick, 2003; Yanay and Benjamin, 2005). Ben Shahar (1993), Drory, Posen, Vilner and Ginsburg (1998) and Rubinstein (2004) have discussed the response to disaster situations by social work departments. A number of key factors have been identified in developing social work disaster responses: the involvement of social workers with other hospital clinical departments in coordinated disaster exercises; training all social workers in the disaster response and their roles and tasks; 24 hour on call procedures; undertaking therapeutic interventions with disaster affected persons; providing information; facilitating contact between disaster affected persons and their families; practical assistance to ensure safety and comfort; establishing the hospital facility as a place of safety as well as medical care; developing procedures for managing staff rosters; establishing effective referral processes and relationships with community organisations providing follow-up services; counselling and other intervention with hospital staff; providing ongoing support structures for staff; undertaking operational debriefs and small group work; and building in flexibility and a culture of participation in the department. Shahar also emphasised the importance of being aware of the theoretical basis underpinning the practice intervention.

## *EARLY INITIATIVES*

The development of the Australian hospital social work response has emerged from the convergence of two phenomena: the establishment of 'twenty-four hour, seven day a week' social work cover in hospitals, and the emergence of a new social work role in forensic medicine.

In 1989 the Social Work Department at Westmead Hospital began to provide a twenty-four hour service to the hospital. As well as being on duty during the normal day shifts, an 'emergency after hours social worker on call,' was also available (Webb, Roberts, and McLaughlan, 1986; Truswell, Blyth, Kendall and Shipway, 1988; Hemp, 1996; Larson, 1997).

At the same time, a social work position was established in the Department of Forensic Medicine and was located in the mortuary. The Westmead Mortuary is one of two city morgues in Sydney and has a coroners court co-located with it.

Coroners' courts were introduced in feudal England over 800 years ago and their core function has changed little over this time. In essence, the coroner's role is to establish, in the public interest, the causes of sudden, suspicious, violent or unnatural death.

The social work role in the Department of Forensic Medicine, included the following activities: providing families with assistance and information about post mortem procedures, the forensic and coronial process establishing the cause of death, inquests, organ donation, and viewings of the deceased. Social workers also provided assistance with funeral arrangements, victim of crime information, grief counselling and referral to community services for follow up intervention.

## *RELOCATING SOCIAL WORK*

These two developments moved social workers from being 'day workers' to being part of the 'core business' of the hospital: a facility that is open twenty-four hours a day, seven days a week. The relationship between the social workers in Emergency, Intensive Care, Forensic Medicine and the After Hours On-Call Service developed quickly, and was based on shared cases, case hand overs, involvement in common issues and job satisfaction derived from crisis intervention work and the 'adrenaline rush' (Coffey, 2001). As a result of these relationships, a new social work team was developing with specific expertise in this area.

Apart from changes in service delivery, these new roles brought with them a significant change in the perception of social workers by other staff. It resulted in the inclusion of social work in many new activities within the hospital.

The main Hospital Disaster Committee invited the Director of Social Work to become a member of the committee, in recognition of the psycho-social care required for disaster affected persons. Social Work became one of several key, functional sites or services in the Hospital Disaster Plan facilitating the hospital's response to the psycho-social needs of all disaster affected persons.

During the early 1990s, a specific Social Work Services Disaster Plan was written for Westmead Hospital that was grounded in the established role carried out routinely by hospital social workers. The plan was consistent with, and modeled on, similar plans established in other countries.

*The Standard Operating Procedure for the Social Work Plan* states:

> The function of the social work service is to coordinate and provide care to relatives and friends of disaster victims. This will include the registration of relatives on arrival at the hospital, the provision of individual psycho-social support for disaster affected persons and bereavement intervention.

In the event of a disaster response being called, social workers were to be deployed to the Emergency Department, Intensive Care Unit, Family Assembly Area, Discharge Lounge, Hospital Wards and the Mortuary (Westplan, 2003). The plan and its implementation were based on the key factors identified by Ben Shahar (1993).

The content of the Westmead Hospital Social Work Disaster Plan includes concise, easy to read descriptions and flow charts of the communication and reporting structures within the hospital during a disaster response, a list of functional sites and the contact details of the site co-ordinators. The Standard Operating Procedures (SOPs) for the social work service are also included. Each functional site has a one page SOP that is included in the main Hospital Disaster Plan so each site can see at a glance the 'larger picture' of the integration of activities.

Role and task cards have been developed for each role within the social work response, for example, role cards have been developed for the Social Work Site Co-ordinator, Emergency Room Social Work Co-ordinator, Family Assembly Area Co-ordinator and After Hours Social Worker should an incident occur then. Each card is set out using the same format and lists the title and function of the role and a list of tasks that the worker needs to undertake when assuming that role. Lessons learned from previous disaster responses indicated that each disaster presents new and unexpected problems. These cards are used as prompts and provide 'a place to start' for workers in a Disaster situation (see Table 1).

The cards have also been photo-reduced to the same size as workers' ID badges and can be attached to the lanyard clip for easy access. The cards are laminated and also have a list of phone numbers on the back that might be useful in the immediate response.

Each member of the Social Work Department involved in the disaster response has a role card including the clerical support staff. The cards help to alleviate the initial anxiety and stress when a disaster page is received. They help focus the workers' attention to a series of tasks while events unfold.

The Social Work Department has a 'disaster suitcase' which is a medium size airline pull bag (on wheels) with zipper compartments. The contents of the bag include: fluoro-coloured vests with 'Social Worker' on the front and back (these are to Australian design specifications for all vests that identify disaster personnel); role cards for all staff deployed; language translation cards; phone numbers and contact lists for the hospital and community services; stationery items including drawing pins, scissors, staplers, tape, board markers; a torch; and a small battery operated radio to listen to media reports that often provide the most up to date information. Two-way communication devices can be provided by the hospital communications center if cellular phones are not functional. The suitcase is a mobile resource that enables social workers to establish a family assembly/information area either within the hospital or off site. The department's clerical staff is responsible for maintaining up to date phone and information lists in the disaster suitcase.

The social workers deployed to the Family Assembly and Information Area of the hospital liaise with the Police Missing Persons Unit to assist in the location and reuniting of family members and disaster victims. In a disaster, the police have responsibility for this task and activate the National Registration Information System (NRIS) which is the primary system used to register and track disaster victims within Australia.

The Social Work Disaster Plan and the contents of the role cards are reviewed regularly and are used in staff training for disaster responses. In particular the Plan is reviewed if an incident has occurred and the Plan has been activated. A recent example is an operational debrief that occurred following a fire in an aged care residential facility in January

## TABLE 1. Examples of Role and Task Cards

---

ROLE CARD:        AFTER HOURS SOCIAL WORKER: INITIAL RESPONSE

LOCATION:        Social Work Department/Emergency Department.

                  The After Hours social worker will only be contacted when a disaster is declared (not for disaster alerts).

REPORTS TO:      Disaster Commander–switchboard extn 58080.

MAIN FUNCTION:  The After Hours Social Worker becomes the Site Co-ordinator for Social Work and Personal Services.

SPECIFIC ACTIVITIES:

- Once contacted by the hospital switchboard, ascertain the details of the disaster from the Disaster Commander (located at the switch). Ask switch who to speak to.

- Contact the Chaplain on call personally and notify of the disaster. Name and number is obtainable from the hospital switchboard.

- Organise a place to meet with the Chaplain on call.

- Contact the Director of Social Work or the Deputy Director of Social Work.

- Come into the hospital.

- Collect and turn on trauma page 08548 from Social Work Department.

- Report to the Site Co-ordinator for the Emergency Department (Senior Nurse Manager or delegate).

ONCE THE AFTER HOURS SOCIAL WORKER COMES INTO THE HOSPITAL THEY ASSUME THE DUTIES OF THE SOCIAL WORK AND PERSONAL SERVICES SITE CO-ORDINATOR (UNTIL RELIEVED BY DIRECTOR OF SOCIAL WORK/DELEGATE).

- Advise the Disaster Commander of the location of the Family Designated Area (FDA).

- Liaise with Security to open up the Education Block (if this is to be the location of the Family Designated Area).

- Liaise with catering to provide refreshment counter in the Family Designated Area.

- Review Role Card for Site Co-ordinator, Social Work and Personal Services and Undertake duties as required.

---

| ROLE CARD: | SOCIAL WORK CO-ORDINATOR EMERGENCY DEPARTMENT |
|---|---|
| LOCATION: | Emergency Department. |
| REPORTS TO: | Site Co-ordinator, Social Work and Personal Services (Director of Social Work) page 27618 Social Work Department extn 56699 and Site Co-ordinator, Emergency Department (Senior Nurse Manager). |
| MAIN FUNCTION: | To allocate and co-ordinate the provision of Social Work service to patients in the Emergency Department. Co-ordinate information flow about patients within the Emergency Department and to external sites such as the Family Designated Area and Social Work Department. |

SPECIFIC ACTIVITIES:

- Allocate social workers in Emergency Department to patients in Emergency Department.

- Ensure social workers follow up patients and relatives, and observers.

- Liaise with Senior Nurse Manager in Emergency Department and Site Co-ordinator of Social Work and Personal Services re situation.

- Liaise with Site Co-ordinator (Director of Social Work) re mortuary arranagements.

- Liaise with ambulance and Police services.

- Co-ordinate with social workers from ICU and wards (ensure relatives are escorted to appropriate wards, ensure that handover is given to appropriate ward social worker).

- Ensure all Emergency Department social workers record all work done in the medical record.

- Deploy, supervise and monitor workloads of social workers in the Emergency Department.

- Co-ordinate list of patients in the Emergency Department and location.

- Liaise with clerical staff re relative information.

- Ensure that an agreed system exists for matching patients and relatives.

- Receive the patient registration card from social workers in the Emergency Department so contact can be made with the patient.

- Receive lists from the Family Designated Area of relatives in the Family Designated Area. Co-ordinate and match these lists. Pass on this information to the social workers working with these patients.

- Liaise with the Police Missing Persons Unit and provide data for NRIS

- Monitor arrival of relatives and ensure they are redirected to the Family Designated Area via escorts and runners.

- Ensure that handover is given to appropriate ward social workers.

TABLE 1 (continued)

ROLE CARD:      CLERICAL STAFF

LOCATION:      Social Work Department 56699

REPORTS TO:      Clerical Co-ordinator reports to the Site Co-ordinator, Social Work and Personal Services.
Clerical Staff report to the Clerical Co-ordinator.

MAIN FUNCTION:      To support the work of the Social Work Department during a disaster response.
To ensure that communication channels are kept open.

SPECIFIC ACTIVITIES:

- Contact the trauma chaplain on call if requested.

- In consultation with the Site Co-ordinator, locate and contact social workers to attend briefing session.

- Assists the Site Co-ordinator to distribute relevant information from the Disaster Suitcase.

- Ensure that channels of communication through the switchboard are kept open.

- Screen calls and direct to appropriate source.

- Assist social workers in the family Designated Area with the registration of relatives and provide other assistance as requested.

- Ensure that supplies of equipment–stationery, forms, pamphlets are available.

- Advise the Site Co-ordinator of any difficulties/changes.

- Keep a list of social workers on duty and area to which they have been allocated and time of commencement of duty.

- Provide access to phones for relatives.

- Assist social workers with information and in contacting other staff.

- Act as runners if requested.

- Ensure that the information lists in the Disaster Suitcase are updated as required.

- Any other duties as requested by the Site Co-ordinator.

2003 that resulted in the elderly residents being evacuated to Westmead Hospital. Social workers worked around the clock to contact family members and find new and suitable accommodation for many residents. The forms used to gather information from disaster victims were tested and modified after this event.

In addition to the regular reviews of the Plan, activities such as continuing education and staff preparation are maintained as part of the annual calendar of department activities. These activities provided a framework within which health professionals respond in each new situation. In addition to the Plan, establishing working partnerships between agencies and professional staff is essential. Social workers, like other health professionals, need to work with people whose work they trust. This provides another foundation for the emergency response.

## A NEW ROLE EMERGES

### Disaster Victim Identification (DVI) Teams

In 1996 Australia established a national Disaster Victim Identification (DVI) team and is party to an international agreement co-coordinated by Interpol (Lyon, France) about how this work should proceed in the event of mass casualties. Disaster victim identification is a very complex, precise and slow process. Successful and correct identification occurs when the ante mortem and post mortem information are a 'mirror image' of each other, that is, there is a complete match. Ante mortem information is collected using a very detailed (nine page) Interpol form. Disaster victim identification also involves other techniques such as finger printing, dental information, medical records of the victim, photography and DNA. Identification by a relative is not relied upon exclusively as this can be incorrect (Edwards, 2001).

### Thredbo Landslide

The relationship between hospital social workers and those in forensic medicine was strengthened further in 1997. Two ski lodges collapsed in a landslide in the ski fields of southern NSW in July 1997 resulting in eighteen deaths. Social workers from Westmead and several other Sydney hospitals were requested to join the forensic counselling team to work with the Disaster Victim Identification Unit and the coroner. The workers were seconded from the hospital on the basis of their experience, skills and training in dealing with trauma and in assisting families with all aspects of bereavement intervention.

The social workers were asked to attend the Missing Persons Unit (MPU) at the Police Operations Command, where arrangements were made for families of those persons missing to be interviewed by police from the MPU in the company of a social worker. Each team was assigned a number of families for the purpose of collecting ante mortem information, providing families with correct information about the details of the disaster, and procedures that would be followed after the retrieval of their relatives from the disaster site. The social workers provided ongoing assistance and support to families.

## *Working with the Coroner/Forensic Medicine: A Clear Role for Social Work*

The role social workers undertake with the coroner in disasters is unique and is not provided by any other professionals. The authority and mandate of the coroner in these situations affirms the social work role with police and with the families of victims. It also assists in the relationship with other disaster services. The role has been tested and reviewed at operational debriefs that have occurred after each disaster. Hospital social workers, experienced in trauma work, are seconded to work with the forensic counselling team for the duration of the response. (The forensic counselling team is made up of social workers that work in forensic medicine as part of their normal duties.) The duties of the seconded social workers at the hospital where they normally work are covered by social workers remaining at the hospital. This level of cooperation and support for social work colleagues undertaking this work has become a feature of the overall response.

## *One Night in Paradise*

On October 12th, 2002 a terrorist bomb blast in the nightclub precinct of Bali's Kuta Beach resort killed over two hundred tourists, eighty-eight of whom were Australian nationals. Many more were critically injured. Bali is a small island to the north of Australia and is a backpacker destination for thousands of young, mainly Western tourists each year. The proximity of Bali to the Australian mainland, and the large number of Australian casualties, resulted in the immediate disaster response being undertaken by Australia in cooperation with Indonesian authorities.

There was a lack of accurate information during the first forty-eight hours about the number of victims and the overall coordination of the disaster response. This was primarily due to the large number of state and federal authorities who became involved as a result of the disaster site being located in another country over which Australian authorities had no jurisdiction. These further complications added to the distress of families trying to find family members (The Age, 15/10/02, 18/10/02; Sydney Morning Herald, 19/10/02; Australian Financial Review, 18/10/02, 21/10/02).

Two social workers from Westmead Hospital joined a team of seven social workers brought together by the Department of Forensic Medicine Sydney. Working closely with the Police Missing Persons Unit and the State Coroner, a social worker and a MPU police officer visited each family to collect ante mortem information. Social workers were allocated to each family and they provided ongoing information, emotional support and practical assistance in the days up to and following the lengthy and complicated process of the identification of victims and their repatriation home.

This work was undertaken by experienced hospital social workers who normally work in the Emergency, Intensive Care and Trauma Units of the hospital. Their skills in crisis intervention, emotional support, practical assistance, and grief and bereavement counselling enabled them to become an integral part of the combined responses of Forensic Medicine, the State Coroner, Police and Health services during the first three weeks after the bombing.

Confirming our well learned lesson that every disaster presents new and different situations, the operational debrief by the team following the disaster focussed on a number of issues including: the number of government departments involved; the lack of official jurisdiction of the site; the slow process of victim identification; media involvement and unsolicited offers of counselling. The disaster site at Kuta Beach was also a crime scene and much of the scene had been disturbed before Australian forensic experts arrived.

The study by Somer et al. (2004) emphasized that the safety of the social workers' loved ones is a priority before any intervention should proceed. Fortunately, in the Bali Disaster no staff members suffered family losses; however, many experienced the personal impact of the catastrophic events.

The work of the Westmead Hospital social workers involved one aspect of the disaster response to the Bali bombing. Social workers in other Australian hospitals, particularly those with burns units, were involved in the ongoing care of the critically injured for many months following the bomb blast.

## CONCLUSION

In reflecting on the development of the Social Work Department's disaster preparedness, and its involvement in a number of disaster responses, it is important to acknowledge the shared learning between international hospital colleagues that has contributed to our 'capacity building' as a health profession, to meet this new and confronting challenge.

The Mt. Sinai Leadership Enhancement Program has nurtured leadership in the social work profession and has encouraged social workers to assume new roles within their health care organisations.

The integration of the social work role into hospital/health disaster plans is one example of how a new role has been forged for the benefit of individuals and service recipients. Social workers have stepped into roles in disaster responses that they have traditionally performed in hospital settings.

Social work intervention, which reflects the suggested approach in the literature, has remained within the framework of dealing with normal reactions to catastrophic events. The intervention also occurs within the framework of professional values to which social work ascribes. Disaster responses continue to be refined and social workers continue to learn from each other, making links with international colleagues, adapting practice to local situations, and individualising care to clients.

International collaboration in programs such as the Mt. Sinai Leadership Program has assisted the development of a critical mass of expertise in this work. Ongoing exchange and scholarship provides affirmation of the work, and support for each other, in this challenging and demanding role.

## REFERENCES

AUSTRALIAN FINANCIAL REVIEW: 'No Relief for the Bereaved' 18/10/2002

AUSTRALIAN FINANCIAL REVIEW: 'Number of Missing Falls' (21/10/2002)

Baker L & Zakour M J (1996) 'A model of disaster response: A public sector and social work education partnership. Paper presented at the CSWE Annual Program Meeting, Washington, DC.

Beck R J & Franke D I (1996) 'Rehabilitation of victims of natural disasters' *Journal of Rehabilitation* 62 (4) 28-32

Ben Shahar I (1993) 'Disaster preparation and the functioning of a hospital social work department during the Gulf war,' *Social Work in Health Care* Vol 18 (3/4) NewYork: The Haworth Press, Inc.

Boes M E (1997) 'A typology for establishing social work staffing patterns within an emergency room' *Crisis Intervention and Time Limited Treatment* 3 (3):171-88

Boscarino J A, Figley C R & Adams R E (2004) "Compassion fatigue following the September 11 terrorist attacks: A study of secondary trauma among New York City social workers *International Journal of Emergency Mental Health* 6 (2) 57-66

Coen J (1997) Thredbo Landslide Disaster Victim Identification (DVI) counselling response. *AASW Newsletter* September Vol 3

Coffey T, Pryor A, & McMahon M (2001) 'The 4am adrenalin rush: A review of after-hours crisis social work service delivery in teaching hospitals' *Visions around the Globe*, 3rd International Conference on Social Work in Health and Mental Health, University of Tampere, Finland July 1-5th, 2001

Dodds S & Neuhring E (1996) 'A primer for social work research on disaster' in C L Streeter & S A Murty (eds) *Research on Social Work and Disasters* New York: The Haworth Press, Inc.

Drory M, Posen J, Vilner D & Ginzburg K (1998) 'Mass casualties: an organizational model of a hospital information center in Tel Aviv' *Social Work in Health Care* 27 (4) 83-96

Edwards M (2001) 'Management of the deceased: Disaster victim identification' presentation at Australian Disaster Medicine Course Sydney. (Chief Inspector Edwards is Chairperson, Interpol International DVI Standing Committee)

Emergency Management Australia (1999) *Disaster Medicine: Health and Medical Aspects of Disasters Manual 2*: Australian Emergency Manuals Series

Fein E & Knaut S A (1986) 'Crisis intervention and support: Working with the Police' *Social Casework* 276-282

Freedman M (1987) 'The continuous traumatic stress disorder; The single therapeutic interview' *Psychology in Society* 8: 46-79

Friis K & Mowll J (2003) *Summary of disaster victim identification counselling response for the Bali disaster* unpublished.

Groner E (1978) 'Delivery of clinical social work services in the emergency room: A description of an existing program' *Social Work in Health Care* 4: 19 -29

Heggar A (1993) 'Emergency room: Individuals, families and groups in trauma' *Social Work in Health Care* 18 (3/4): 161-168

Hemp S (1996) 'Social work services after hours: Developing an on-call program,' *Social Work Administration* 22 (8)

Hicks P (1999) 'The crash of Flight 703: A hospital's response' *Aust NZ Journal Surgery* 69:573-575

Hodge J (2000) 'Responding to mass casualty incidents in the rural setting: A case study' *Australian Journal of Emergency Management* 14 (4):29-32

Irizarry C, Gameau B, Walter R (1993) 'Social work leadership development through international exchange.' *Social Work in Health Care* Vol 18 (3/4) New York: The Haworth Press, Inc.

Itzhaky H & York A S (2005) 'The role of the social worker in the face of terrorism: Israeli community-based experience' *Social Work* 50 (2) 141-149

Jacobs G A & Kulkarni N (1999) "Mental health responses to terrorism" *Psychiatric Annals* 29 (6)

Larson L (1997) 'Days without End' *AHA News* Newsletter of the American Hospitals Association, March 31st.

Lee L & Collings A (2000) 'Sydney hailstorms: The health role in the recovery process' *Medical Journal of Australia* 173 4/18 December: 579-582

Lennox G (1996) 'Effective emergency management: Lessons from the Port Arthur tragedy' Australian College of Health Service Executives Professional Development Program Sydney (unpublished)

Lindemann E (1944) 'Symptomatology and management of acute grief' *American Journal of Psychiatry* 101, 141-148

Newburn T (1993) *Disaster and After: Social Work in the Aftermath of Disaster* London: Jessica Kingsley

Newhill C E & Sites E W (2000) 'Identifying human remains following an air disaster: The role of social work' *Social Work in Health Care* 31 (4) 85-105

Novick J (2003) 'The role of the social workers in the aftermath of the World Trade Center attack' *Home Health Care Management and Practice* 15 (2) 152-156

NSW Health (2001) *NSW HEALTHPLAN*: NSW Health Services Functional Area Supporting Plan. (State Health Publication No (PH) 960098) Sydney

NSW Health (2002) *Effective Incident Response: A framework for prevention and management in the health workplace.* Sydney

Neill J (2001) 'Social workers heed call after attacks' *NASW News* 46 (10) 8-10

Rehr H & Epstein I (1993) 'Evaluating the Mount Sinai Leadership Enhancement Program: A developmental perspective' *Social Work in Health Care* Vol 18 (3/4): 147-159 The Haworth Press, Inc. NY

Reyes G & Elhadi J D (2004) 'Psychosocial interventions in the early phases of disasters' *Psychotherapy: Theory, Research, Practice, Training* 41 (4) 399-411

Rubinstein, E (2004) 'The social work role in mass casualty events: An Israeli hospital experience' Key Note Address at Westmead Week: *Health Professionals Working with Mass Casualties: Shattered Lives* (August 25th-27th) Westmead Hospital Sydney

Sherraden M S & Fox E (1997) 'The Great Flood of 1993: Response and recovery in five communities' *Journal of Community Practice* 4 (3) 23-45

Somer E, Buchbinder E, Peled-Avram M, & Ben-Yizhack Y (2004) 'The stress and coping of Israeli emergency room social workers following terrorist attacks' *Qualitative Health Research* 14 (8) 1077-1093

SYDNEY MORNING HERALD: 'The Long Journey Home from Blast's Horrific Injuries' (19/10/2002)

The AGE: 'The Distressing Task of Tracing the Victims–Identifying victims may take months–Relatives provide DNA samples to help identify missing people' 18/10/2002

Truswell S, Blyth J, Kendall S & Shipway P (1988) 'In the eye of the storm: Crisis intervention in hospital' *Australian Social Work* 41 (1): 38-43

Van Ommeren M, Saxena S & Saraceno B (2005) 'Mental and social health during and after acute emergencies: Emerging consensus' *Bulletin of the World Health Organisation* 83 (1) 71-6

Webb F, Roberts R F & McLaughlan S (1986) *After Hours Bereavement Counselling at Parramatta Hospitals*, Report to the Bereavement Counselling Working Party: Westmead Hospital Archives, unpublished.

Westmead Hospital (2003) *Westplan: Westmead Health Disaster Management Plan,* Westmead NSW
Yanay U & Benjamin S (2005) 'The role of social workers in disasters' *International Social Work* 48 (3) 263-276

## Web Sites

American Red Cross
*http://www.redcross.org*

The Federal Emergency Management Agency–FEMA
*http://www.fema.gov/*

Emergency Management Australia
*http://www.ema.gov.au*

# Academic-Practice Partnerships in Practice Research: A Cultural Shift for Health Social Workers

Lynette Joubert, DLitt et Phil

**SUMMARY.** Academic-practice partnerships in practice research support health social workers in engaging in research that is embedded within their practice. This shift in culture enables social workers to join in a health service discourse that is increasingly data-driven and focused on effective practice and demonstrated quality of care for patients. The mentoring model is described as enabling practitioners to superimpose research skills onto existing practice skills. An academic-practice research collaboration can reduce the distance between research and practice, contribute to a body of knowledge for health social work and promote health social workers as "research focused practitioners." *[Article copies available for a fee from The Haworth Document Delivery Service: 1-800-HAWORTH. E-mail address: <docdelivery@haworthpress.com> Website: <http://www.HaworthPress.com> © 2006 by The Haworth Press, Inc. All rights reserved.]*

Lynette Joubert teaches in the School of Social Work at the University of Melbourne and is Research Consultant in the Aged Care and Allied Health Directorate, St. Vincent's Health, Melbourne (E-mail: ljoubert@unimelb.edu.au).

The author would like to acknowledge the support of her health social work colleagues: Sonia Posenelli, Rebecca Power and Maureen McKinerney from St. Vincent's Health, David Nilsson from Western Health, Jane Miller from the Royal Children's Hospital, Millissa Fromer from Melbourne Health and Glenda Bawden from Southern Health. The author also acknowledges the work of Prof. Irwin Epstein who continues to inspire us.

[Haworth co-indexing entry note]: "Academic-Practice Partnerships in Practice Research: A Cultural Shift for Health Social Workers." Joubert, Lynette. Co-published simultaneously in *Social Work In Health Care* (The Haworth Press, Inc.) Vol. 43, No. 2/3, 2006, pp. 151-161; and: *International Social Health Care Policy, Programs, and Studies* (Ed: Gary Rosenberg, and Andrew Weissman) The Haworth Press, Inc., 2006, pp. 151-161. Single or multiple copies of this article are available for a fee from The Haworth Document Delivery Service [1-800-Haworth, 9:00 A.M. - 5:00 P.M. (Est). E-mail address: docdelivery@haworth press.com].

Available online at http://swhc.haworthpress.com
© 2006 by The Haworth Press, Inc. All rights reserved.
doi:10.1300/J010v43n02_10

**KEYWORDS.** Academic practice partnership, collaboration, practice research, mentoring model, research focused practitioner.

Health social workers are increasingly being asked to practice not only in relation to practice wisdom, but to make decisions based on effectiveness and demonstrated quality of care. A new terminology has been added to the health social worker's vocabulary that reflects this cultural shift. The terminology includes terms such as "outcomes," "benchmarking," "pathways of care," "key performance indicators," "quality assurance," "accountability" and "evidence based practice." These terms relate to the activities that drive the current development, implementation, and evaluation of health services. The shift to data-driven expectations of the role of social work in changing systems of health care is part of a more general evidence based discourse in health, and has increased the need for collaborative, practitioner-initiated exploratory, monitoring and evaluation research. This poses a research challenge for health social work.

Academic-practitioner practice research partnerships offer health social work practitioners and their academic colleagues the opportunity to develop collaborative research activity that encourages reflection, contributes to a data base for social work practice and supports social work in joining a research focused, evidence based discourse with their allied health, medical and nursing colleagues.

The School of Social Work at the University of Melbourne has developed a mentoring model of practice research collaboration that is focused on supporting practitioners in developing rigorous research projects from within their own practice or from available data collected as part of a routine hospital service. The collaboration is focused on "learning through doing" and education about research design and process occurs through individual and group mentoring. The feedback of clinical outcomes serves to enhance social work performance and to introduce program change. Other gains reflect the outcomes achieved from clinical services becoming the basis for further study. These include the development of papers for presentation locally and internationally, as well as the preparation of work for publication. This interactive style of learning is interspersed with formal teaching around requested topics. The initiative has been strengthened by the participation of social workers inspired by their association as visiting scholars in the Mt. Sinai Medical Centre exchange program in New York, as well as the subsequent visits of Mt. Sinai practitioners and academics to

Melbourne. This continuing fruitful exchange has offered Melbourne health social work an example of ways in which academia and practitioners can collaborate around issues of mutual concern and acted as a catalyst in the development of collaboration in response to local need.

## BACKGROUND

The demographic shift to an ageing population has resulted in a general shift in health care from treatment to prevention, mortality to morbidity due to chronic illness, and from the management of external threats such as infection and injury, to internal threats such as negative behaviors related to smoking, stress, poor diet and a sedentary lifestyle. This shift is reflected in the 4 national research priorities for Australia, announced by the Prime Minister in December 2002. Research priority number 2 focuses on the prevention, promotion and maintenance of good health across the life span, with particular reference to the young and the elderly, and with a focus on allied health participation: *"research in prevention will emphasize interdisciplinary research"* and *"There is also a need to draw on multi-disciplinary approaches that include research contributions from the social sciences and the humanities."*

The focus on the importance of the interrelationship between the social sciences and the humanities with health has become increasingly recognised, and quality and timely health service delivery includes a focus on psychosocial, functional and behavioral factors. These complex systemic issues have been subjected to a culture of health service delivery, where decisions are made on evidence of suitability and quality, and where treatment effectiveness and cost-effectiveness need to be justified by valid data. Berger (2000) talked about the changing expectations of the role of social workers within evidence based systems of health care. These are reflected in the need to justify intervention effectiveness and cost-effectiveness, with quality assurance dependent on measurable outcomes, and consumer interests and satisfaction with care, influenced by process and outcome evaluation of services. Social workers, advocating for consumer interests, are dependent on studies monitoring and comparing different models of service delivery to motivate for change within health services. The need for health social work to engage in practice based research becomes obvious as practitioners seek to make a credible and valued contribution within a data-driven health care culture.

The organizational benefits for social workers to engage in practice research are balanced by individual, vocational benefits. These were described in a focus group run by the author in 2003 after social workers had participated for one year in an academic practice research partnership. Social workers emphasized professional development and the acquisition of new skills such as data base management, research design, evaluation models and data analysis, which translated into practice and program development. In addition they experienced opportunities to present to colleagues both within social work and interdisciplinary forums, as resulting in increasingly satisfying and respectful dialogue with health care professionals. This had led in some instances to changes in work place procedures. On a personal level they developed increased enthusiasm and motivation for practice, with resulting beneficial outcomes for staff retention. They felt strongly that research opportunities should be listed in the advertisements for social work positions, and cited the active support of both social work and health service management as a critical factor in the shift to a research based culture.

Prof. Irwin Epstein described the key components of a practice research partnership in an address delivered as a Miegunyah Scholar at the University of Melbourne in 1994. These included the open exchange of ideas across institutional and national boundaries, quality practice-based education and continuing education, support structures that promote practice-based research within social work departments and across disciplines, support structures that promote practice-based research by linking the university and social agencies, intra-mural and interdisciplinary accountability structures and leadership roles, serving as models and sources of inspiration. The partnerships developed in Melbourne have drawn on the example of the practice-academic partnership model developed at New York's Mount Sinai Medical Centre. They have attempted to foster reflection amongst health social workers, promote a research culture in social work departments in health services and strengthen integrated inter-professional practice rather than fragmented, silo based, discipline specific health care. These have been supported by the ongoing participation of Prof. Epstein in workshops held in Melbourne on practice based research. In addition, the author has engaged with Prof. Epstein in collaborative mentoring across social work departments, highlighting the possibilities and accessibility of practice research as core "business" in health social work.

Previous studies have shown that collaboration is a complex intervention with multiple components, including process innovation and product innovation. This can result in institutional development and change (Lawson 2004). Most academic practitioner partnerships are focused on programs offering both practice and research placement opportunities for student training. These in turn support practitioners in conducting research, and improve the likelihood of staff participation in research projects (Hall, Jensen, Fortney, Sutter, Locher and Cayner 1996). An educational practice initiative from a school of nursing in Western Australia (Downie, Orb, Wynaden, McGowan, Zeeman and Ogilvie 2001) was felt to have bridged the theory-practice gap with the practice research undertaken contributing to best practice outcomes. The most valued outcome of the collaboration was felt to be the pursuit of research to support clinical practice. Another nursing academic-practice partnership resulted in an annual research and research utilization conference, a series of research roundtables, talks with nurse authors and a Website (Caramanica, Maljanian, McDonald, Taylor, MacRae and Beland 2002). It was felt that the sustained collaboration encouraged more rapid dissemination of research findings into practice, enriching nursing practice and ultimately benefiting patient outcomes.

While there are many nursing and medical initiatives reported in the literature, there is a lack of information on academic-practice partnerships in health social work. An exception is the work of Christ, Siegel and Weinstein (1995) who described the establishment of a research unit as an integral part of a hospital social work department. The evolution of the relationship between the clinical and research staff was characterized by four different phases, which included curiosity, competitiveness, cooperation and collaboration. There was an overall positive effect on the professional practice of staff, who displayed increased academic rigour and productivity although some staff remained unconvinced of the value of the effort. Simarlily, Hall, Jensen, Fortney, Sutter, Locher and Cayner (1996) reported on the value of strengthening both practice and research with the development of collaborative student training programs which included research projects in practice specialties, helped clinicians conduct research, provided students with practical research experience within a clinical setting and increased the likelihood that both staff and students would participate in research.

Collaborative partnerships offer the opportunity for interdisciplinary learning as was found in an initiative undertaken in a geriatric setting (Reuben, Yee, Cole, Waite, Nichols, Benjamin, Zellman and Frank 2003). Four organizational factors were found to be essential in the establishment of collaboration. These included organizational readiness to implement the innovation, the relationship between the academic and clinical organization, the tangible and intangible sources of support at multiple levels within the organization and the administrative and organizational requirements for team training programs. We have found that the research partnership is dependent not only on institutional administrative support, but in particular the support of the social work manager in motivating the health service and social workers to participate in the initiative. Once staff are involved in the practice research mentoring process, this gains a momentum of its own and the shift to research focused practice becomes an accepted process in the department. Randall (2003) emphasized the need for sustained commitment, authentic collaboration and a shared belief in each other as essential to the creation of a "knowledge that works" (p. 125).

## THE PROCESS OF THE PRACTICE RESEARCH MENTORING PARTNERSHIP

The practice research collaboration starts with an "idea" reflecting the practitioner's insight, skill and interest. This is the beginning of an interesting process of conceptualization into a research design, implementation, analysis and dissemination. The focus is on a research process integrated within the demands of the social worker's practice. This necessitates a careful consideration of both the time that it will take to complete the process and the need to complete additional work within a busy work day. As a result, mentoring around the feasibility of the design and the use of existing documentation collected as part of routing practice, either retrospectively as in data-mining (Epstein 2002) or prospectively, become important issues to work through, implement and analyse. The process is on reflective practice, but re-ordered objectively as far as is possible within the rigor of a research methodology. This is in contrast to a more conventional research approach where the process begins with a hypothesis and the researcher seeks the practice environment to explore the question. This latter approach has the luxury of a focus on research alone, a focus on evaluating an opportunity to modify a situation and compare outcomes usually with and without the modification, or undertaking a qualitative exploration of a research question. There is a freedom of research purpose.

In contrast, practice based research with practitioners who have little or no experience of either research design or process, is focused on moving from practice wisdom and passionate interest in an issue, to a research question and process. The challenge within the mentoring relationship is to balance the demands placed on the practitioner in their workplace with research rigor.

This is an applied research context and researcher and mentor must seek out methodologies that are innovative, and access the broader systemic issues that impact on quality care and outcomes. There are certain core values that need to be acknowledged in this process. The first is that no research project is too small to be insignificant to the practitioner who will now have the opportunity to present data on their practice, not only within their immediate professional group, but to their health colleagues or on a more extended conference platform. The second value is that the research process is not a race against time, and research methodologies need to be chosen that allow for flexibility. These could include integrated quantitative and qualitative methodologies, focus groups, ethnographic approaches, grounded research, program logic and data-mining, outcome evaluation, exploratory studies concerning complex issues impacting on health, and factors contributing to effective recovery and disease management.

We have found an increasing interest from health social workers in Melbourne to participate in practice based research. When asked to rate themselves on a scale of 10, ranging from 0 (no interest) to 10 (very high interest), they consistently positioned themselves at 8 and above. In contrast, when asked to rate their knowledge about research on a similar scale from 0 (no knowledge) to 10 (excellent knowledge) the ratings fell to between 5 and 7. This discrepancy can prove to be a powerful barrier to social workers feeling confident to participate in research. We feel that this can be attributed in some instances to a formal education in research methodology that appears unrelated to the practice issues with which they are confronted. In addition, social workers cited a fear of working with numbers, the need to have a detailed understanding of research methodology before attempting research, a fear of presenting in public and the distancing of the research process from everyday practice, as additional barriers to engagement in practice research. The extent to which practice research is embedded in existing practice enables social workers to move to including research as integral to departmental culture.

The shift to a practice research focus can be conceptualized as a shift from the skill base required for practice–

Integrated knowledge of theory and practice

Direct practice skills

Insight into social work practice as it relates to health service delivery

Ability to observe and assess

Ability to record

Ability to analyze and discuss

to a skill base required for practice research.

---

Integrated knowledge of theory and practice

Direct practice skills

Insight into field of practice as it relates to health service delivery: ***Development of a research area, question and design***

Ability to observe and assess

Ability to record: ***Data entry or collation***

Ability to analyze and discuss: ***Analysis of quantitative and qualitative data***

Ability to write clearly: ***Formal report and presentation writing***

---

The mentoring process supports the social worker in applying a research lens to their practice by superimposing practice research skills onto existing practice skills. This reduces the distance between research and practice and assists in a smooth transition from practice issue to research question. The social worker gains confidence in moving to a research question that is grounded in practice wisdom, of passionate interest and relevant to the health service. The mentoring input provides support in developing a methodology, implementing a research process, and in the analysis and discussion of results.

We have found that most practice research designs in health social work can be broadly conceptualised into three main categories. These are outcome evaluation, program evaluation and quality assurance. The following examples of practice research projects undertaken as part of the academic-practice partnership illustrate the three categories and the diversity of issues being researched.

### *Outcome Evaluation*

In an outcome study carried out by the social work manager of an integrated care program at St. Vincent's Health, Melbourne, data-mining was used as a methodology to explore the outcomes of an integrated care program, in responding to the complex problems presented by patients presenting frequently at emergency (ED). The data-mining methodology used in the research process provided the opportunity to use available data routinely collected by team members as part of their practice and entered into an information management database. As a result, the data collection for the purposes of the program evaluation did not intrude on services being offered or on the privacy of patients. It was an efficient method of collecting a sample (N = 94) which was the total population seen by the program over a period of six months.

The research process was divided into three phases. In Phase 1 a retrospective consecutive sample was selected from the program database using a data collection audit tool, which defined the data to be generated from the database. This generated a report highlighting the number of presentations and admissions for one year pre- and post-recruitment into the program, length of stay in ED, reasons for presentation (these included homelessness, substance use, disability and aged care problems) and demographic information. In Phase 2 the data was descriptively analysed, which identified a number (12% of the total population) of "outliers." Outliers were identified by the fact that their number of presentations and admissions had continued to increase (> 5) after being recruited into the program and despite receiving care co-ordination services. Once the outlier sub-group had been identified we developed a questionnaire to use in data-mining of their hospital files. The questionnaire focused on the reasons for presenting at emergency, whether there was consistency in the issues presented, the intervention offered by the ALERT team and access of community services. In Phase 3 we hoped to be able to "add meaning to the quantitative measures" mined from the hospital database in Phase 1 of the research process. The results suggested that within a consecutive sample, there were a sub-group of patients with multiple and recurring issues who did not respond to the usual care coordination intervention offered by the integrated care program, but needed an intensive continuing case management approach to care. They were a minority group, but highly significant in terms of their impact on the outcome evaluation of such programs in the emergency department.

An immediate outcome of the evaluation was the implementation of intensive long term case management based on client needs and service collaboration within the integrated care program. The work was presented locally and written for publication.

## Program Evaluation

A program evaluation of a newly integrated allied health structure was driven by the social work manager, who had been instrumental in the development of the innovation at St. Vincent's Health and mentored by the academic partner. The aims for the integrated allied health structure included realizing opportunities for improvements across the care continuum, the need for a workable and cost effective structure for allied health and promotion of the organization's integration agenda.

In the two years since the restructure was completed, the Allied Health Heads of Departments had shown leadership in promoting the integration agenda with a shift from an integration structure to an integration culture. There was a growing group identification and acceptance of the purposes of the group. The methodology for the evaluation attempted to capture the cultural change as well as being user-friendly in encouraging maximum participation across allied health practitioners. Invitations were extended to managers and staff to be part of a voluntary, confidential process where they would complete individual questionnaires. Focus groups were held immediately following their completion.

The analysis of the combined quantitative and qualitative data set collected through the process of reflexive evaluation demonstrated that while the impact of the restructure had been excellent at the higher and middle management levels, structures, processes and jointly established goals needed to be created for junior levels of staff to identify with. The content analysis of qualitative data clearly indicated the need for increased and more meaningful channels of communication to be established at junior levels of staff. This was in contrast to the high levels of satisfaction with the quality of clinical care, and a strong commitment to the values of the organization. The evaluation has promoted a continuing agenda of integrated allied health practice.

### Quality Assurance

In an attempt to improve the quality of the service offered to the children of mothers with breast cancer in acute care, a social worker mentored within the academic-practice partnership data-mined ward files (Epstein 2002) and audited the responses of hospital staff to including children and families in their management of mothers with breast cancer. These were found to be minimal. She conducted a triangulated needs study, which explored the needs of patients and families in relation to services that could be provided from an acute health care setting. The practice research project produced significant outcomes. The ward documentation was changed to include a genogram, a family and child friendly room was incorporated onto the ward, and the social worker presented for the first time at an international conference with subsequent publication of the work as a textbook chapter (McKinerney and Joubert 2005).

## CONCLUSION

Academic-practice research partnerships offer health social workers the opportunity to incorporate research from within their own practice. We have found that this has resulted in a cultural shift in social work departments to the integration of research as a priority for social work managers. Randall (2002) spoke of the need for stronger and more credible relationships between practitioners on the one hand and researchers on the other.

The academic-practice research mentoring model aims to integrate practitioner and researcher in one person–a research focused health social worker.

## REFERENCES

Caramanica L. Maljanian R. McDonald D. Taylor SK. MacRae JB. Beland DK. (2002) *Journal of Nursing Administration.* 32(1): 27-30.

Christ GH. Siegel K. Weinstein L. (1995) Developing a research unit within a hospital social work department. *Health and Social Work.* 20 (1): 60-9.

Downie J. Orb A. Wynaden D. McGowan S. Zeeman Z. Ogilvie S. (2001) A practice-research model for collaborative partnership. *Journal of the Royal College of Nursing.* 8(4): 27-32.

Epstein I. (1995). Promoting reflective social work practice: Research strategies and consulting principles. In E.J. Mullen & P. Hess (Eds.), *Practitioner-Researcher Partnerships: Building Knowledge From, in and for Practice.* New York: Columbia University Press.

Epstein I. (2001). Using available clinical information in practice-based research: Mining for silver while dreaming of gold. *Social Work in Health Care.* 33(3/4), 15-32.

Epstein I. Blumenfield S. (Eds.) (2001). *Clinical data-mining in practice-based research: Social work in hospital settings.* Binghamton, NY: The Haworth Press, Inc.

Hall JA. Jensen GV. Fortney MA. Sutter J. Locher J. Cayner JJ. (1996) Educating of staff and students in health care settings: Integrating practice and research. *Social Work in Health Care.* 24(1/2): 93-113.

Lawson H. (2004) The logic of collaboration in education and the human services. *Journal of Interprofessional Care.* 18(3): 225-37.

Mizrhi T. Abramson JS. (2000) Collaboration between social workers and physicians: Perspectives on shared care. *Social Work in Health Care.* 31(3): 1-24.

Randall J W. (2002) The Practice Research Relationship: A Case of Ambivalent attachment? *Journal of Social Work.* Vol 2, No 1, 105 (122).

# Outcomes from the Mount Sinai Social Work Leadership Enhancement Program: Evaluation and Extrapolation

David Nilsson, DSW
Anna Wellington-Boyd, BSW

**SUMMARY.** This article presents an overview of outcomes from the Mount Sinai Leadership Enhancement Program as identified by previous program participants from Melbourne, Australia. These are categorised into: (1) Personal/professional, (2) Intra-organisational, (3) Inter-organisational, and (4) International outcomes. Two illustrative examples are provided of international outcomes demonstrating how the ongoing commitment of Professor Epstein has extended and embedded the principles of practice-based research in Melbourne, and how the over-riding principles of the program have been applied by participants in establishing collaborative relationships with colleagues in our neighbouring South-East Asian region. *[Article copies available for a fee from The Haworth Document Delivery Service:*

David Nilsson is Allied Health Manager–Social Work, Western Health Network, Melbourne, Australia; Honorary Fellow, School of Social Work, The University of Melbourne; and Associate Fellow, Australian College of Health Service Executives (E-mail: David.Nilsson@wh.org.au). Anna Wellington-Boyd is Senior Social Worker/Trauma Stream-Leader, The Alfred Hospital, Melbourne, Australia.

[Haworth co-indexing entry note]: "Outcomes from the Mount Sinai Social Work Leadership Enhancement Program: Evaluation and Extrapolation." Nilsson, David, and Anna Wellington-Boyd. Co-published simultaneously in *Social Work in Health Care* (The Haworth Press, Inc.) Vol. 43, No. 2/3, 2006, pp. 163-172; and: *International Social Health Care Policy, Programs, and Studies* (ed: Gary Rosenberg, and Andrew Weissman) The Haworth Press, Inc., 2006, pp. 163-172. Single or multiple copies of this article are available for a fee from The Haworth Document Delivery Service [1-800-HAWORTH, 9:00 a.m. - 5:00 p.m. (EST). E-mail address: docdelivery@haworthpress.com].

Available online at http://swhc.haworthpress.com
© 2006 by The Haworth Press, Inc. All rights reserved.
doi:10.1300/J010v43n02_11

*1-800-HAWORTH. E-mail address: <docdelivery@haworthpress.com> Website: <http://www.HaworthPress.com> © 2006 by The Haworth Press, Inc. All rights reserved.]*

**KEYWORDS.** Leadership enhancement, outcomes evaluation, international implications

The Mount Sinai Social Work Leadership Enhancement Program was originally established in 1989 to offer leadership development opportunities for Israeli Hospital Social Work Directors. Australian social work health-care managers were also included from 1990 after a Melbourne social work academic, Catherine James, successfully advocated for our inclusion. This three-month program has generally been offered on an annual basis and includes up to four participants (although the number of participants has varied on occasion).

Up to this time there have been a total of twenty-seven Australian participants. Whilst Australia-wide participation has been encouraged, the majority of participants have come from the state of Victoria where the organising committee (the Australian Association of Social Workers International Continuing Education Committee–AASW ICEC) is based (sixteen from Victoria; four from New South Wales; two each from South Australia and Queensland; one each from Tasmania, Australian Capital Territory and Northern Territory).

For comprehensive background details of the program, readers are referred to Drs. Rehr, Rosenberg, and Blumenfield's informative (1993) article, "Enhancing Leadership Skills Through International Exchange: The Mount Sinai Experience."

In summary, this 10-12 week program consists of approximately four weeks of orientation providing an overview of relevant departments, services, and programs within the context of the medical center and the city of New York. The structured adult learning model then provides open access to an extensive range of documentation, personnel and meetings. Participants also pursue an individual learning program (e.g., developing specialist areas of knowledge, research projects, program initiatives, etc.). While immersing themselves in the life and culture of Mt. Sinai Medical Center and of New York City, participants are exposed to a range of leadership models and provided with instruction on practice-based research principles and academic/practice partnership development.

The key aims of the program are to enhance participants': Leadership capabilities; Knowledge and skills to implement quality programs;

Ability to assess and improve programs; Ability to conduct applied studies; Improvement of social health policy; Develop cost effectives of service programs (Rehr et al., 1993, p. 22).

One of the primary outcomes of this program has been to promote a more lateral approach within leadership and management thinking in regard to social work program development and management in healthcare. This spans all levels of management practice including micro (being the individual), meso (including organisational practices) and macro (which ultimately incorporates an international perspective and issues relating to globalisation).

There are a number of important reasons for evaluating the outcomes of the program for past participants. Firstly, for reflective practice purposes it is of interest to the participants themselves to review the benefits accrued from the program and the effects upon their subsequent professional development. It is also important to members of the Australian ICEC committee that they continue to review the outcomes of the program so that they can correctly advise future participants of the particular benefits to be gained, and more importantly to provide recommendations to the Mt. Sinai organisers as to which aspects of the program were of the greatest value in meeting the intended goals and resulted in beneficial outcomes.

Indeed, Rehr et al. (1993) note that, "Follow-up evaluation of change at individual, departmental, institutional, and community levels would be sought at later periods when visitors had returned home and would assist ongoing program development" (p. 26). This article summarising information from presentations at the 2004 Doris Siegel Colloquium aims to partially fulfil that goal.

The genesis of the presentation at the Doris Siegel Colloquium was also inspired from Dr. Blumenfield's informative key-note address on *Collaboration in the New Era* at a symposium held in Melbourne in October, 2000. Her address resonated with the experiences of those present who had participated in the Leadership Enhancement Program and inspired them to re-evaluate their progress.

The structured evaluations which inform this article took place in two parts. For reasons of convenience relating to access to participants, they were limited to previous participants solely from Victoria in Australia.

The initial evaluation was undertaken by the second author in 1994. This included a review of all available documentation and in-depth semi-structured interviews with five previous program participants. This was a wide-ranging evaluation which covered the participants' expectations prior to, experiences during, and post participation.

The second evaluation was jointly undertaken by both the authors in March 2000 and included a small survey and a focus group discussion relating to participants perceived outcomes of the program. This included a total of eleven program participants.

## INDIVIDUAL PROFESSIONAL AND PERSONAL DEVELOPMENT OUTCOMES

Respondents identified numerous individual professional and personal development outcomes that resulted from the program. Firstly, all returnees noted that a significant feature of the program had been their recommitment to their social work identity and the profession in general after witnessing the strong, inspirational role-models within the senior management team of the Mount Sinai Social Work Services department. Participants also frequently reported returning feeling 'rejuvenated' and having increased levels of motivation to tackle difficult issues within their various work environments.

Many respondents noted that their individual leadership skills had further developed from implementing the *Take Charge Survival Strategies* as were presented by Dr. Blumenfield at the 2nd International Conference on Health and Mental Health. These strategies included the foci of *maintaining perspective*, *developing population-based services*, and *adding value* and *taking ownership*.

Another result of having participated in the program has been that approximately half of the Victorian participants have gone on to enrol in further post-graduate study.

Several participants also noted the tangible flow-on effects in terms of career enhancement after having gone on to secure more senior positions since returning from the program. Indeed, one participant secured a key health management role in Melbourne while still actually on the program. Her interviewers appeared quite impressed at her selection for, and participation within, this esteemed program.

## INTRA-ORGANISATIONAL OUTCOMES

At an intra-organisational level, the implementation of Dr. Blumenfield's *Take Charge Survival Strategies* has led to a greater level of proactivity within service development initiatives, the development of strategic partnerships (particularly through inter-disciplinary collaboration), and has reportedly resulted in raising the profile of social work services within participants agencies and being seen to add value to organisational activities.

There has also been a notable sharing of leadership knowledge from the program participants within their own organisations (and also between organisations). Some of this has occurred through role-modelling, mentoring and supervision processes. The ripple effects of learning have also occurred through the collaborative efforts such as those described in the *Survival Strategies* implementation. This has been described by Cath James as *distributive leadership.*

Another important outcome from the program has been the development of practice-based research efforts. An integral component of the Leadership Enhancement Program is the model of practice-based research taught by program consultant, Irwin Epstein (Helen Rehr Professor of Applied Social Work Research, Hunter College). The benefits of such an approach have been realised through implementation by several program returnees within their organisations. For example practice-based research programs have been instituted at the Cancer Council of Victoria, The Early Psychosis Prevention and Intervention Centre, and the Royal Children's Hospital of Victoria.

## *INTER-ORGANISATIONAL OUTCOMES*

The practice-based research efforts have also developed into more formal academic/practice partnerships for several organisations. Most of these have developed with the University of Melbourne and, significantly, all have involved past Mt. Sinai Leadership Enhancement Program scholars. These partnerships are continuing to grow in strength and can be seen to be a tangible outcome of the program.

Additionally at an inter-organisational and professional level, past program participants have maintained an active and influential role within several of the AASW Special Interest Groups. These include the *Health Social Work Directors Group*, the *Victorian Oncology Social Workers Group*, and a *Practice-Based Research Interest Group*. These are further examples of *distributive leadership* creating change through ripple effects.

As a sub-committee of the *Health Social Work Directors Group*, ICEC holds regular forums to promote the program and further international collaborative efforts. Past program participants have also taken up opportunities of presenting on the program and its beneficial outcomes at numerous conferences.

## INTERNATIONAL OUTCOMES

The Leadership Enhancement Program returnees have been active not only in presenting at a national level, but also internationally, and have also been instrumental in the development of international conference initiatives such as the International Conferences in Health and Mental Health. These notably evolved out of the Leadership Enhancement Program initiative at Mount Sinai.

Another important outcome of participation in the program was identified as the development of international "connections." The concept of an international "community" of social work health-care managers has been described as being of particular value to previous program participants in terms of being a source of both additional collegial support and informational resources.

The development of these international collegial relationships has also resulted in a number of professional visits to Australia by key Mt. Sinai staff. The first of these was by Helen Rehr (Professor Emeritus, Mt. Sinai School of Medicine) in 1985. In 1998 Melbourne hosted the Second International Conference on Health and Mental Health which resulted in a number of Mt. Sinai staff visiting Melbourne. Susan Blumenfield (Mt. Sinai Social Work Director) returned in 2000 followed by Virginia Walther (Senior Assistant Social Work Director, Mt. Sinai) in May 2002 and in March 2005, Nancy Cincotta (Mt. Sinai Oncology Preceptor) also undertook visits to Melbourne and Sydney. Each of these senior staff provided guest lectures, and consultations with senior health care staff.

The model of international exchange of knowledge from the Mt. Sinai program has also been directly influential in the establishment of the *Victorian Oncology Social Workers Group*. This group have begun an exchange program with like-minded colleagues in the United States in order to share relevant knowledge and experience within their specialist area of practice.

## EXTENSION OF PRACTICE BASED RESEARCH

As previously described, there have been a number of enhanced research, educational and professional development opportunities that have flowed from the connections made through the program but one of the most tangible and useful examples has been the ongoing commitment of Professor Epstein in providing specialist consultancy on practice-based research development. Professor Epstein has continuously made himself available not only by email and phone but has undertaken an extensive series of visits to Australia (May/June 1994, July 1998, June/July 1999, March 2001, January 2003, June 2003, April 2004, June 2005).

Professor Epstein's first visit in May 1994 was as *Miegunyah Scholar* at *The University of Melbourne*. His *Miegunyah Address* was entitled *Integrating the challenge and challenging the integration of research and social work practice* and outlined his vision for the development of practice-based research and furthering academic-practice partnerships. The key themes outlined in that address over a decade ago have formed a solid framework for the developmental work that he has gone on to promote through his ongoing contact.

The key themes outlined in that address included the needs for: (1) Open exchange of ideas across institutional and national boundaries; (2) Quality, practice-based research education and continuing education; (3) Support structures that promote practice-based research within social work departments and across professional disciplines; (4) Support structures that promote practice-based research by linking the academy and social agencies; (5) Intra-mural and interdisciplinary accountability structures that engage professionals in pursuits that include but transcend self-interest and self-promotion; and (6) Leadership (i.e., individuals who serve as models and inspirations).

Through Professor Epstein's contributions during that visit, Australian health social workers were exposed to new possibilities for research and professional development. There was a heightened understanding of social work as an international profession similar to that of medicine.

Correspondence back to Mt. Sinai at that time notes "the ripple effect . . . and groundswell of cultural change via program returnees" and "Professor Epstein's role as a catalyst . . . providing inspiration and momentum . . . helping envisage social work within the international context"; ". . . an invaluable contribution. I feel he has put us about five years ahead in terms of winning the hearts and minds of the social workers here about the value of practice research. Equally, he has really lifted our profile and credibility within the research community here."

During his visits to Australia, Professor Epstein has provided numerous consultations, lectures, keynote presentations and workshops at hospitals, health services, universities, and for government officials. He has provided many specialist consultations to six different health care networks within Victoria as well as to others in South Australia, New South Wales and Queensland. His work at *The University of Melbourne* has included consultations with the *Course Advisory Committee*, lectures for undergraduate and post-graduate students, consultations on thesis development, facilitation of faculty workshops, consultation on the development of the MSW (Health) degree and on the formation of a collaborative *Social Work Academic-Practice Health Research Consortia.*

Over the succession of his visits, Professor Epstein's work has expanded to include a greater focus on inter-disciplinary approaches to research. This began during his 1998 visit in providing consultation to the multi-disciplinary team at the *Early Psychosis Prevention Centre* and continued through his facilitation of a series of workshops in 2001 for the *Allied Health & Nursing Research Group* at the *Royal Children's* Hospital. These workshops included participants from Nursing, Occupational Therapy, Physiotherapy, Play Therapy, Psychology, and the Child Protection Unit. The 2001 visit also included multi-disciplinary consultations across the *Youth Drug & Alcohol Services* at the *Western Health Network.*

The inter-disciplinary approach continued in the January 2003 visit with a practice-based research lecture for multi-disciplinary staff at *North-West Mental Health Service* followed by workshop consulting on staff research projects and through a series of research consultations at the *Alfred Hospital* and at the *Young Persons Health Service* to develop plans for research and evaluation of activities.

As a result of the overwhelming positive responses to these multi-disciplinary consultations, Professor Epstein was invited to provide the keynote address for *Practice-Based Research for Allied Health Professionals: A skills oriented symposium* in June 2003.

Professor Epstein's continuing commitment and leadership has personified the values and principles of the Mt. Sinai Leadership Enhancement Program. His continued inspirational input has tangibly increased research development not just for social work, but also a range of other allied health disciplines.

## *SINGAPORE NETWORK DEVELOPMENT*

Another international outcome that owes its inception to the innovative Mt. Sinai Leadership Enhancement Program has been the development of professional and educational links between health social workers in Melbourne and our south-east Asian neighbours, most notably in Singapore. This has resulted in several exchange visits and the establishment of some educational and professional development placements. The Singapore Melbourne Health Social Work Network was formally established in 2002.

The network was originally established to provide an easily accessible conduit for enquiries about visiting Melbourne and to promote collegiate contact and friendships between social workers in Singapore and Australia. It has resulted in seven Singaporean health social workers undertaking work-place based "attachments" in Melbourne, enrolments of Singaporean student in post-graduate courses at *The University of Melbourne*, and several collaborative academic-practice visits to Singapore.

The key aims and elements of the Network are described in the subsequent article by Jane Miller. The Network holds monthly meetings in Melbourne which are quite informal and provides opportunities for meeting with visiting social workers from Singapore. They are able to connect with Australians at a social level and to present on aspects of their work. Australians also report on their visits to Singapore. Academic-practice partnerships are promoted through the strong support that the Network receives from *The University of Melbourne School of Social Work*. The Network maintains communication through use of its extensive email contact list consisting of approximately 100 members in both Australia and Singapore.

This Network has been built on the basic principles of the Leadership Enhancement Program and the ideals of internationalism that it embodies. The developmental processes employed have aimed to use the social work concepts of networking and community development to respond to varying requests and needs identified. The outcomes achieved thus far by the Network are viewed as a exciting beginning and it is anticipated that these connections will further strengthen and provide *distributive leadership* outcomes similar to those achieved from the Mt. Sinai Leadership Enhancement Program.

## CONCLUSION

In conclusion, the findings indicate that the numerous outcomes from the program are indeed multi-layered and inter-connected at the personal, professional, organisational, and international levels. They can also be seen to be continuing to develop as the "global-picture" of health management continues to change in unpredictable ways.

The previous participants all agree that the program has been successfully improving social work health-care management in Victoria primarily through enhancement of the individual participant's leadership skills, and secondarily through the practices of *distributive leadership*.

It is also clear that exchange on an international basis is incredibly valuable for professional development at a senior level. It can be seen that it can act as a catalyst for broader educational, research and professional development.

It is important to note the limitations on outcomes that were also identified through the evaluation process. It appears that there has been limited success with the particular goal of enhancing development of new programs. This may in part be due to the prevailing political environment in the state of Victoria over the last decade during which there was a particularly conservative government with regressive policies. The entire health-care sector suffered rolling financial cuts during that time which is likely to have affected the potential for development of new programs. Nevertheless, that aspect of the program remains an achievable goal.

Overall, however, it is concluded that the program serves as an excellent model for international contribution and collaboration within the profession.

## REFERENCE

Rehr, H., Rosenberg, G., & Blumenfield, S. (1993) Enhancing Leadership Skills Through an International Exchange: The Mount Sinai Experience. *Social Work in Health Care*, 18(3/4),13-33.

# Skills, Bravery, Courage, and Foolhardiness: Seventy-Five Years of Social Work in Health Care in Melbourne, Australia

Jane Miller, MSW, MAASW

**SUMMARY.** The lessons from the history of health social work in Melbourne, Victoria can be extrapolated to social work in other parts of Australia and internationally. Based on consultation with social workers, archival material and personal reflections this article traces 75 years of health social work in Melbourne and Victoria within the context of the prevailing social influences. The profession, which was started by local opinion leaders and public demand, is now well established. Initially Australians looked to Britain to guide the new profession, but by the latter part of the twentieth century they increasingly looked to the USA. Many challenges still face health social work. Sharing of knowledge and experience will strengthen social work locally and internationally. *[Article copies available for a fee from The Haworth Document Delivery Service:*

Jane Miller is Chief Social Worker, Royal Children's Hospital, Flemington Road, Parkville, Melbourne, Victoria 3052, Australia (E-mail: jane.miller@rch.org.au).

The author wishes to thank the following for their generosity in provision of factual information, recollections and advice: Glad Hawkins, Linette Hawkins, the late Wendy Weeks, Catherine James, Kathy Sanders, Sonia Posenelli, Archives St. Vincent's Hospital, Elizabeth Steeper, Archives AASW Victorian Branch, Jan Fook, Lynette Joubert, Bronwyn Hewitt (Archives Department, Royal Children's Hospital), Elery Hamilton Smith, Helen Rehr, and Jane Sullivan.

[Haworth co-indexing entry note]: "Skills, Bravery, Courage, and Foolhardiness: Seventy-Five Years of Social Work in Health Care in Melbourne, Australia." Miller, Jane. Co-published simultaneously in *Social Work in Health Care* (The Haworth Press, Inc.) Vol. 43, No. 2/3, 2006, pp. 173-191; and: *International Social Health Care Policy, Programs, and Studies* (ed: Gary Rosenberg, and Andrew Weissman) The Haworth Press, Inc., 2006, pp. 173-191. Single or multiple copies of this article are available for a fee from The Haworth Document Delivery Service [1-800-HAWORTH, 9:00 a.m. - 5:00 p.m. (EST). E-mail address: docdelivery@haworthpress.com].

Available online at http://swhc.haworthpress.com
© 2006 by The Haworth Press, Inc. All rights reserved.
doi:10.1300/J010v43n02_12

*1-800-HAWORTH. E-mail address: <docdelivery@haworthpress.com> Website: <http://www.HaworthPress.com> © 2006 by The Haworth Press, Inc. All rights reserved.]*

**KEYWORDS.** Health, social work, history, Australia, international

## INTRODUCTION

Social work is still a relatively young profession. While it does date back to the late 19th century in some countries (USA and Britain for example), in others such as Singapore, local training of social workers did not commence until after the Second World War (Wee, p. 9). The initial impetus for social work training and the perspectives of early leaders vary in different societies. In Singapore, for example, the early influence was the London School of Economics (Wee, p. 8), whereas in Finland health social workers evolved from the work of the 'social nurses' in the 1920s. Australia's early influences were British, but by the latter part of the twentieth century health social work looked more to the United States of America.

This brief history of the development of health social work in Melbourne (in the state of Victoria) traces development from its origins in hospitals in 1929 to today's well established generic profession with six university training courses in this Australian state alone.

The chains of choice and circumstance in the development of health social work in Victoria have influenced its status and style today.

## OVERVIEW

In seventy-five years health social work in Victoria has grown from an 'experimental training course' (O'Brien & Turner 1979, p. 6) graduating around four students per year to work in hospitals to a strong generic profession which graduates over 200 students per year from six universities in Victoria (Hawkins et al., 2000, p. 35)

In this article the words almoner, medical social worker and health social worker will all be used to refer to practitioners in the field of health social work. The original British name for hospital social workers was 'almoner.' The role was seen as an extension of the Charity Organisation Society's enlightened 'scientific' charity work (O'Brien & Turner 1979, p. 6). Medical social worker was the common terminology from the 1960s. The common usage became health social worker in the 90s.

Social Work is a product of its context and a systems based profession. Accordingly a history of social work needs to be viewed within its social context. The practice of health social work has been shaped not only by prevailing social attitudes but also by social needs. For convenience I have divided this history into four arbitrary phases: Establishment 1929-50; Professional consolidation–demand outstrips supply 1950-70; Exponential growth of profession–turmoil 1970-1990; Supply exceeds demand–higher profile 1990-2003.

## PHASE 1: ESTABLISHMENT 1929-1950

### Social Environment–Key Features

This period covers the Great Depression, the rise of Fascism in Europe, the Second World War and its aftermath, which included mass immigration from Europe. During this period the racist White Australia Policy was in place (preventing immigration of people of non-European background). Aboriginal Australians were largely ignored, generally denied citizenship and were regarded as members of a dying race. The depression, which ended with the Second World War, resulted in high unemployment and severe poverty. Itinerant men travelled Australia looking for work. Families were forcibly evicted from homes for non-payment of rent. Until the late 50s homeless Melbourne people were housed in former army camps on inner city parklands. There was limited government welfare provision.

Without modern antibiotics and vaccines, Tuberculosis was a serious and often fatal disease requiring months or years of quarantined hospitalisation in one of the three state TB sanatoriums. There were also regular polio epidemics, which killed many and left others permanently disabled with 'infantile paralysis.' Hospitals charged means tested fees.

### The Impetus to Establish Almoning in Victoria

The move to establish almoning in Victoria came from influential public servants, doctors and female charity workers. Organisational supporters included the Charity Organisation Society, the Australian Red Cross Society and the Melbourne Hospital's Social Service Bureau (O'Brien & Turner 1979, p. 20). Miss Agnes McIntyre of St. Thomas' Hospital London established the first Australian Almoner Department at the Melbourne Hospital in 1929. The Victorian Almoners were the first Victorian (and Australian) social workers.

### Commencement of Almoner Training

The Victorian Institute of Hospital Almoners commenced training the first Melbourne students in 1931. They undertook a fifteen-month (later two-year) course, which involved a strong in-service component. They attended a mixture of University and Workers' Education Association lectures as well as receiving tuition from Miss McIntyre at the Melbourne Hospital. Almoners' work was practical: assessing patients' ability to pay for medication, appliances, finding homes for patients' children, and arranging convalescent care (O'Brien & Turner 1979, p. 26). By the end of this period today's more intrapsychic approach had commenced. The shift was more toward the patient and their perception rather than 'doing to.' At the Third National AASW conference held in Adelaide in August 1951, Miss H. James noted that she would 'place emphasis on the word "understanding," especially as it applies to the patient himself and how he feels about his situation, rather than how the almoner feels about it' (James 1936, no page numbers).

At the point of winding up in 1950, the Victorian Institute of Hospital Almoners published a small booklet (author anonymous) summarising its work. It states that upon the establishment of the Institute 'it was immediately evident, however, that the need for a training course for general social work was basically even more urgent and important than the need for a training course for medical social work only' (1950, p. 6). A public meeting was convened at the Melbourne Town Hall. There was unanimous agreement on the need for a social work training course. The popularly endorsed committee that resulted from this meeting commenced general social work training of the first five Victorian trained generic social workers in March 1933. The generic course was transferred to the University of Melbourne in 1941. Until its closure in 1950 the Institute of Almoners provided strong support to the generic course (The Origin and Development of Medical Social Work in Victoria 1950, p. 6).

The move to generic social work training was in step with approaches in the United States and Britain. However, the Institute had some trepidation about handing over medical social work training to the generic University course: 'The only remaining reason for its [the Institute's] continued existence would be to safeguard and foster the interests of medical social work and its practitioners in Victoria' (The Origin and Development of Medical Social Work in Victoria 1951, p. 9). The responsibility to ensure this was handed to the Australian Association of Hospital Almoners (Victorian Branch). Despite the careful planning of the Almoners' Association the interests of medical social work did not remain a paramount concern for the profession during the ensuing rapid change and expansion in the profession as a whole.

During the first part of this phase an average of 5 or 6 almoners completed training annually. Between 1947 and 1950 there was approximately double this number (O'Brien & Turner 1979, p. 41). Figures for generic social workers are not available for all years. However, in 1942, 12 and in 1948, 19 social workers graduated from the University of Melbourne (Malseed & Schuyers 1973, p. 142). In the whole of Australia there were 95 qualified social workers employed in 1941 (Lawrence 1965, p. 89).

## PHASE 2: PROFESSIONAL CONSOLIDATION 1950-1970

The demand for social workers was increasing. At the beginning of this phase the annual graduating class from the University of Melbourne (School of Social Studies) numbered 14 (in 1952), and by the end it was 78 (Malseed & Schuyers 1973, p. 118). In 1958, 148 social workers were employed in Victoria and just five years later in 1963 there were 248 (Malseed & Schuyers 1973, p. 98).

### Social Environment: Key Features

In this period Melbourne underwent radical change. Australia's post war immigration scheme resulted in increased population and cultural diversity particularly with the arrival of many non-English speaking families.

New suburbs sprang up. The Victorian Housing Commission pursued an active 'slum clearance' policy, moving long established inner urban families to the Housing Commission Estates in outer suburbs or the new prefabricated high rise flats.

This era was politically conservative, fuelled by Cold War fears of the spread of Communism. Federal government social security provision remained limited, with charities playing many of the roles now played by government. The State Government provided some of the welfare benefits subsequently provided by the Federal Government. The Victorian Council of Social Services published a Directory of Social Services for Victoria, a slim volume.

## Education

The Diploma of Social Studies at the University of Melbourne, the only training available in Victoria, was a strong three-year vocational course. It included six field placements preceded by numerous visits of observation to agencies. By graduation students were well socialised into their profession. It was common to combine the Diploma with a Bachelor of Arts, resulting in four years of undergraduate study. At this time no postgraduate studies were offered. Students who wished to continue to study at the Masters level had to look to other faculties or overseas.

However, a specialist medical social work stream was taught by practitioners.

## Hospitals as a Workplace for Social Workers

The Victorian Hospital and Charities Commission oversaw the activities of both hospitals and the voluntary sector. As this suggests public hospitals had their origins in charity and retained a charitable ethos. Senior medical staff, the equivalent of today's medical consultants, were called 'honoraries' as they were unsalaried. Hospitals employed debt collectors who visited patients at home.

By now medical social work departments existed in the major teaching hospitals but rarely in the geriatric or country hospitals. Freud's work was influential. Social work took on an increasingly psychological approach.

Apart from doctors and medical scientists, social workers were virtually the only staff who had university degrees. Occupational therapy, speech pathology and physiotherapy practitioners were still trained by their own special institutes. Nurses were trained on the apprenticeship system. In my opinion, this gave social workers a certain confidence and authority.

The names of the departments gradually reflected the change from 'almoner' to 'social worker,' although many were still called 'Almoner Departments' into the 60s.

Social relationships tended to be more formal than today. Social workers and students wore white coats. Students, supervisors, social workers and clients all addressed each other by formal titles: Miss, Mr., or Mrs. In some hospitals social workers were barred from reading or writing in medical records. Social recording was exacting and in general the passive voice was used. Referrals were usually formal written referrals from doctors and case finding was not common.

## Workforce Issues

Systemic discrimination against women in the workforce had an impact on this predominantly female profession. Issues included lack of equal pay, ineligibility for superannuation (if married), and unavailability of childcare. Most women gave up work for a substantial period of time, if not permanently, after having children.

There were insufficient social workers to meet demand. Various schemes were developed to attract social workers to particular organisations. These included bonded scholarships from the Victorian Hospitals and Charities Commission and the Mental Hygiene Authority. For the broader social work field the new Victorian Social Welfare Department sent its employees, mainly male, to be trained at the School of Social Work (Melbourne). There was a general view that the profession needed to attract more males if it was to succeed (Lawrence 1965, p. 198).

## Professional Issues

The Australian Association of Social Workers (AASW) Victorian Branch was very active at this time. Senior members visited the University to recruit new members directly from the graduating classes. The fact that the Federal AASW office was located in Melbourne strengthened the professional presence.

The Victorian Branch had an active medical social work group. The minutes of the meeting of 11th June 1964 to examine the rules for membership of the group illustrate their concerns about standards and professional expertise. They moved that membership of the group should be confined to: 'Persons who are members of the AASW and are either qualified medical social workers or have practiced in a clinical medical setting under the direction of a qualified medical social worker for a period of not less than two years' (AASW (Vic) Newsletter 11.6.64).

The ensuing discussion included concern that if membership were restricted to those who met their criteria The Medical Social Work group would lose the opportunity to teach and mentor those less qualified.

The first forty years of social work in Victoria was marked by a steady growth in a small and tight-knit professional group. Knowledge and work practices had evolved in keeping with changes in society's demands and social attitudes. There was naturally occurring collaboration between academic social workers and practitioners (partly because the pool of experts was so small that practitioners had to be called on to teach). The Victorian Branch of the AASW provided a forum for exchange of ideas and promotion of the profession. It was both the social workers' union and the professional association. The small numbers in the profession and the fact that almost everyone had been trained at the same school of social work led to cohesiveness.

## PHASE 3:
### EXPONENTIAL GROWTH OF THE PROFESSION–
### TURMOIL 1970-1990

The 1970s was a time of unprecedented growth of the social work profession in Victoria (see Figure 1): the annual number of graduating social workers increased threefold, from 73 in 1969 (Malseed &

FIGURE 1. Total Social Work Graduates in Victoria 1929-1994 (includes almoners)

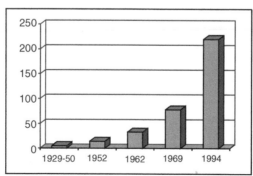

Combined data from O'Brien & Turner (1979), Malseed & Schuyer (1973), Hawkins (2000)

Schuyers 1973, p. 141) to approximately 230 per year in the early 90s (Hawkins et al., 2000, p. 37).

The result of the exponential growth of social work was that for approximately 20 years the field was imbalanced towards social workers who were still learning their profession. A group of experts is needed to lead best practice in any profession. (Fook Ryan and Hawkins' study of professional expertise details the key features of social work expertise (p. 186) which is comprised of a set of complex and hard won set of skills, values, theory and understanding which take some years to develop.)

In the following section I shall show that while by the end of the phase the supply of social workers did meet demand in Victoria, the period of undersupply had resulted in lack of continuity in social work departments in hospitals, employment of unqualified staff in social work roles. Erosion of pay and conditions may also have discouraged graduates from choosing a career in health social work.

## *Social Environment: Key Features*

This period was characterised by widespread dissent in Australia as in Western society generally. This included mounting opposition to the war in Vietnam and the birth of the second wave women's movement. Key gains (nationally) included: legal abortion, generally available childcare; equal pay, female entitlement to permanency in the public service and to superannuation regardless of marital status; and availability of home loans to single women. Improved contraception resulted in improved career opportunities for women who could now plan parenthood.

The Whitlam Federal Labor Government (1972) introduced many reforms. A universal free health care system, Medibank (later Medicare) was introduced. All doctors in hospitals became salaried; all Australians became entitled to free hospital treatment. In 1974 the federally funded community health program commenced. Federal Social Security entitlements were widened to provide a universal safety net.

From the late 70s onwards, the concept of rights for minority groups was accepted, resulting in a range of state and federal equal opportunity and human rights legislation. Rights frameworks and the concept of 'social justice' became generally accepted.

Deinstitutionalisation commenced with the closure of most major total institutions. In the health arena deinstitutionalisation was seen as one of the ways to 'normalise' disability (Wolfensberger, 1972).

## The Hospital as a Workplace for Social Workers

Social workers gradually shed their white coats. Clients and social workers addressed each other by given names. The distance between patient ('supplicant') and professional ('expert') was breaking down. The more radical social workers espoused patients' rights and particularly during the International Year of the Disabled Person (1981) worked collaboratively with the burgeoning disability rights groups. Family therapy became popular with social workers.

## Workforce Issues

The AASW (Victorian Branch) took a leadership role in addressing concerns about undersupply of social workers. In conjunction with the Institute of Applied Economic Research of the University of Melbourne it conducted a needs study which was published in 1973.

Findings included that the number of social work positions was expanding rapidly. Between 1968 and 1972 the number of new social work positions increased at the rate of 40 jobs per year (Malseed & Schuyers 1973, p. 117). This doubled the number of social work positions in Victoria. They predicted (p. 132) there would be a 164% increase in hospital social work positions in the ensuing decade. They also predicted that in the next decade (to 1982) between 786 and 1089 additional social work positions would be created in Victoria (across all fields).

Despite the growth in the numbers of social workers there was a lack of strong and consistent social work leadership at senior levels in hospitals at this time. For example, at the beginning of this phase (early 70s) there were still three general hospitals in Melbourne that did not have social work departments at all. In addition social workers were rarely employed in either geriatric or country hospitals. Commonly, lack of availability of trained social workers led to the employment of welfare assistants (Malseed & Schuyers 1973, pp. 45-47).

Toward the end of the phase James (1988) surveyed all Victorian hospital social work departments (73 in all) and found both lack of continuity in the role and a significant number of non social workers occupying head of social work department positions.

Two-thirds of department heads (22 out of 73) had qualifications such as welfare, nursing and 'other tertiary,' qualifications (James 1988 p. 20). Almost a quarter (24%) of rural heads of department had less than one year of service (in the position). Length of service in the period studied was typically between 4 and 9 years in the city hospitals but her report notes that in the year after she conducted her survey (1988) over half of the 13 heads of the large and special function teaching hospitals had retired or resigned (James 1988, p. 21).

Examination of the minutes of the Health Social Work Directors' Group Meetings confirms Ms. James' findings. The membership of heads of hospital social work departments in the decade from 1981 to 1991 had turned over completely. Two of the 1991 members of the group were still in the group in 2001.

## Education

Malseed and Schuyers' (1973) report resulted in the establishment of additional schools of social work in Victoria. The second Victorian social work course was established in 1973 at Preston Institute (PIT, later known as Phillip Institute); Monash University commenced in 1974 and Latrobe University in 1976. This brought diversity to the teaching of social work in Victoria (Weeks 1993; Weeks n.d.).

During the 80s a number of rural campuses and distance education courses were established to help address the undersupply of social work in rural areas.

Post graduate social work education became available. The first to offer this was Melbourne University which commenced their Masters program in the early 70s, followed over the ensuing five years by Monash and Latrobe Universities.

## Industrial Issues

Two major industrial changes affected the practice of professional social work in Victoria: the rise of related occupational categories (such as welfare officer, youth worker, community development worker) and the creation of the Australian Social Welfare Union.

The lack of supply of social workers in Victoria had led to the development of related occupational categories and for at least a decade the welfare industry could not have functioned without them.

The AASW which combined the role of professional association and union for social workers was then faced with a dilemma. Many of the new occupational categories in the welfare field were without industrial awards. It was in the interests of both social workers and the new occupational groups to have one union to negotiate for everyone.

It was decided to separate the industrial and professional roles of the AASW. Thus, the Australian Social Welfare Union was created by a narrow vote in 1975. (Hawkins, G 2003) Under the management of the ASWU in Victoria, wages of social workers declined significantly in comparison with equivalently qualified colleagues in hospitals. It seems probable that the poor wages and conditions offered to social workers in Victorian hospitals militated against attracting and retaining excellent staff as equally interesting and better paid work could be obtained in local government, State and Commonwealth government departments.

## Professional Issues

Some of the theoretical debates that were influential in the 70s were: critiques of the 'medical model'; a radical anti professional critique; Ivan Illich and 'iatrogenic illness' (Illich 1997); and feminism and the status of women in social work (Nichols 1974).

During the 70s the AASW Victorian Branch still maintained close contact with the membership. It facilitated grass roots social action from practitioners by auspicing social workers wishing to present submissions to a range of government inquiries. The work of the Regional Accommodation Team Services Group in the Melbourne eastern suburbs hospitals is one example (Goodman, Nichols & Gould 1983, p. 27).

In the early 70s the Head of Social Work at St. Vincent's Hospital initiated the Senior Social Workers in Hospitals Group as a special interest group of the AASW Victorian Branch. This group has met regularly to the present day. It is currently known as the Health Social Work Directors' Group. The purpose of the group was to share ideas and information, offer support and work collaboratively on matters of mutual interest.

The minutes of 20.12.83 captured something of the flavor of the group under 'Correspondence In' from the group's founder, Marjorie Awburn, on her retirement, she is quoted as saying she had found the group one of 'useful and cohesive men and women, outstanding for the excellence of their intellectual and theoretical social work knowledge and skills, their bravery, courage and foolhardiness, exceptional optimism and possibly bloody mindedness (for such is the stuff of which social workers in hospitals are made!)' (AASW 1983).

## PHASE 4: SUPPLY OUTSTRIPS DEMAND–
## OPPORTUNITIES FOR CONSOLIDATION
## AND PRACTICE EXCELLENCE 1990-2004

### Environment

The beginning of this phase when a very conservative state government came to power was a difficult time for the health sector and social workers. The period was characterised by a highly ideological economic rationalist philosophy which included a push to privatization, forced tendering by hospitals for their own existing services, hospital amalgamations, attempts to reduce the power of unions and the award system, introduction of individual short term employment contracts, significant staff cuts and retrenchments. Social workers involved themselves in industrial action with stop work meetings and union rallies. It was a threatening environment in which debate was stifled. 'Politically correct' became a term of abuse. In Victoria the introduction of Casemix Funding (Hickie 1994) was used to drive cost cutting. While a more liberal government subsequently came to power some of the changes introduced have remained.

### Workforce Issues

The main change in the workforce in this period and up to the present was the likelihood that new social work graduates would not necessarily be employed in a job designated 'social worker,' although they would find employment in the traditional social work sectors of health and welfare. Research into the early employment paths of newly graduated social workers carried out in 1995 and 1996 found that 'overall, it can be said that employment opportunities in the welfare sector in Victoria are no longer primarily occupationally defined . . . Vocation-specific qualifications including social work, only accounted for 12% of positions' (Hawkins et al. 2000, p. 35). However, in hospitals employment has continued to be based on professional qualifications and categories and social workers are usually employed in distinct social work departments.

In many hospitals social workers have developed formal alliances with related professions such as physiotherapy and occupational therapy. By the end of this phase in many hospitals Allied Health Departments or Divisions were developed. This is a marked change from the previous decade where most heads of department reported to medical directors (James 1988, p. 23).

## Education

Two more schools of social work were commenced: Victoria University of Technology 1991 and Deakin University 1993. During this period the PIT course was subsumed by Royal Melbourne Institute of Technology (RMIT) as a result of the merger between the two institutions.

In 2003 the University of Melbourne commenced the first Victorian specialist Masters in Health Social Work. In its first year it had 28 enrolments. There is a strong practice content in this course which was designed by an academic and a practitioner and is guided by a reference group of senior practitioners who regularly teach in this course.

## Industrial Issues

This period saw the regaining of parity of wages and conditions of employment of social workers in Victorian hospitals with other Allied Health workers with equivalent qualifications (physiotherapists, etc.) through the move from the lagging Social and Community Services Award to the Allied Health Award (Health Services Union of Australia no 3 Branch). Wages and conditions of social workers in the health sector now compared favorably with other fields of social work. For example, this is the only award in Victoria where social workers are paid a generous 'higher qualifications allowance' for a post graduate diploma or degree.

## Professional Issues

The influence on health social work in Victoria of the Mount Sinai Social Work Leadership Enhancement Program has been important. This program has now been undertaken by fourteen Victorian senior social workers. This three-month program provides the opportunity for two Australian and two Israeli social workers each year to participate in a specially designed adult learning program in one of the world's leading hospital social work departments. Research into the experience of returnees has shown that individuals feel validated, inspired and return to their workplaces with a new sense of vision and purpose (Rehr, Rosenberg & Blumenfield 1993, p.13; Nilsson 2004).

Close collegiate relationships have been developed with a number of the Mount Sinai social workers. In particular Professor Irwin Epstein from Mount Sinai and Hunter College New York has provided inspirational leadership for development of practice based research in health social work in Melbourne.

More formal promotion of academic practice partnerships has also resulted from exposure to the Mount Sinai model. For example, a number of Melbourne's major teaching hospitals have formal agreements with the University of Melbourne in relation to both student and research units.

Inextricably linked with the Mount Sinai program is the triennial International Conference on Social Work in Health and Mental Health Care. This conference series commenced in Israel in 1995, was held in Melbourne in 1998, Finland 2001 and Quebec 2004. It was born out of the professional relationships between Australian, American and Israeli social workers created through the Leadership program.

Eighteen Victorian social work practitioners and academics gave papers at the Israel conference, 153 attended the Melbourne conference, the majority making presentations and over 20 presented at both Finland and Quebec. Four Melbourne social workers are on the International steering committee of this conference series.

The development in 2004 of a Health Special Interest Group of the Victorian Branch of the Australian Association of Social Workers is evidence of the renewed vigor of the health social work sector.

A quiet change in 2004, the introduction of eligibility of certain registered private practice social workers for reimbursement for their services by the National Health Insurance Commission through the Federal Department of Health and Ageing may result in an increase in the number of social workers in private practice (Johnston 2004). Unlike the situation in the USA, most private health funds at present do not reimburse for social work consultations, whereas they do for psychology.

## *DISCUSSION*

Today the large number of qualified social workers in the workforce, the availability of post graduate education and the existence of a cohort of expert social workers who were the graduates of the 70s to provide leadership and expertise augurs well for the profession's future in the health sector.

The combination of a ready supply of highly educated graduates and the improved industrial conditions will assist in the attraction and retention of well qualified social workers in hospitals. This is not to deny the complexity of factors which keep good social workers in hospitals. As pointed out by Pockett (2003), factors which encourage retention of good social workers include such features as providing an environment where the social worker can be both strongly integrated into the core business of their unit while able to exercise professional autonomy.

Nevertheless, the perception of a *glass ceiling* which limits social workers but not medical and nursing staff will need to be addressed. Alternative, flexible career paths will need to be found in hospitals. This may include academic/practice appointments, combining hospital work with a private practice (a common approach in the USA), enhancing work satisfaction with opportunities for research and teaching or promotion into generalist hospital roles such as discharge planner, case/care manager or other middle management roles which draw on core social work skills and experience.

Despite the gains made, health social workers have no cause for complacency. Challenges include: increasing pressure for demonstration of outcomes and the demand for an evidence base for interventions; the trend in some hospitals to devolve social workers into medical programs or allied health departments where they are managed in interdisciplinary teams by non-social workers; and challenges from related professions such as nursing, psychology or 'counselling' to work in the traditional core areas of social work.

There are more serious challenges for the social work profession as a whole. At the time of writing there are significant tensions within the Australian Association of Social Work regarding the roles and rights of the state branches versus the national association. Some members of the Western Australian Branch have seceded and established a competing organization. Reform is clearly needed. The Association plays a key role in promoting the profession, negotiating with government, setting standards for entry to the profession, and producing the national journal and conference, but it cannot do this effectively without the confidence of members and a high proportion of membership of practicing social workers.

There is a need for more Australian social work journals. Australian Social Work, the journal of the AASW, is too general to be able to provide a forum for debate for health social workers (and the many other specialist areas of the profession.) Advances in Social Work and Welfare Education and Women in Welfare Education are the only other local professional journals.

Australia needs to be alert, as we follow the path of American social work, about the threats (as well as opportunities) of social workers moving into private practice. This can well enhance the profession's status, but as pointed out in Unfaithful Angels: How Social Work Has Abandoned its Mission (Specht & Courtney 1995), it is important that it does not skew the profession away from its mission to the *disadvantaged and its commitment to social justice..*

## CONCLUSION

Over 70 years health social work has demonstrated an ability to adapt to changing societal needs and expectations. In that time expertise and knowledge in the profession as well as public profile has changed and grown. In a debate on the future of health social work at the Melbourne International Conference in Social Work in Health and Mental Health (1998), Professor Ron Feldman, Dean of Social Work at Columbia School of Social Work argued that social work would survive because it is a 'chameleon profession.'

Cross national comparison which is facilitated by such initiatives as the International Conference on Social Work in Health and Mental Health, the journal Social Work in Health Care and by opportunities for inter country professional exchanges will enrich practice in individual countries wherever they are on the journey to establishment of the social work profession.

Perhaps, above all, Marjorie Awburn's words of 1983 should be remembered: as well as bravery, courage and foolhardiness, what social work leaders internationally will continue to need will be 'exceptional optimism and sheer bloody mindedness.' This makes an innovative leader.

## REFERENCES

Australian Association of Social Workers (1964) *Newsletter: Medical Social Work Group, June Special Meeting, 11.6.64: Examination of Rules of Membership of the Medical Social Workers' Group.* Victoria Australia

Australian Association of Social Workers (1986) *Senior Social Workers Inter Hospital Group Minutes of Meeting, July.* Victoria Australia

Australian Association of Social Workers (1991) *Senior Social Workers Inter Hospital Group Financial Members as at 23/8/91*

Australian Association of Social Workers (1981) *Senior Social Workers Inter Hospital Group, Minutes of Meeting at Prince Henry's Hospital Tuesday 15th December 1981.* Melbourne Australia

Fook, J, Ryan, M, & Hawkins, L (2000) *Professional Expertise: Practice, theory and education for working in uncertainty.* England. Whiting & Birch Ltd.

Goodman, H, Nichols J, Gould, J (1983) "Action" *Social Work in Action: The Politics of Practice: Proceedings of the Eighteenth National Conference of the Australian Association of Social Workers, NSW* 27-32

Hawkins, L, Ryan, M, Murray, H, Grace, M, Hawkins, G, Hess, L, Mendes, P, Chatley, B (March 2000) *Supply and Demand: A Study of Labour Market Trends and the Employment of New Social Work Graduates in Victoria?: Australian Social Work* March 2000 Vol. 53 No 1 p. 35

Hawkins, G (2003) *Background to Formation of Australian Social Welfare Union (unpublished account by the inaugural Federal Secretary of the Australian Social Welfare Union)*

Hickie, J B (1994) "The Challenge for Clinicians" *The Sixth National Casemix Conference Proceedings' "Casemix for Clinicians"* Commonwealth Department of Human Services and Health Canberra Australia.

Illich, I (1977) *Limits to medicine: Medical nemesis: The expropriation of health,* Harmondsworth, NY, Penguin.

James, C (1988) *Social Work in Public Hospitals of Victoria: A preliminary overview and discussion paper* (unpublished)

James, C (1987) "An Ecological Approach to Defining Discharge Planning in Social Work" *Social Work in Health Care,* Vol. 12, No. 4, 1987

James, H (1951) 'Medical Social Work' 1951 *Proceedings of the AASW Third National Conference Adelaide 24-28 August 1951 (no page numbers)*

Johnston, A (2004) *Update of the New Medicare Benefits Item–Allied Health Services* AASW National Bulletin: Newsletter of the Australian Association of Social Workers vol 14 Issue 2 November-December 2004

Lawrence, RJ (1965) *Professional Social Work in Australia,* Canberra, ANU

Malseed, E & Schuyers, G (1973) The Demand for and Supply of Professionally-Trained Social Workers in Victoria, 1972 to 1982, Institute of Applied Economic Research, University of Melbourne

Miller, J (2001) "The Knowledge, Skills and Qualities Needed for Social Work in a Major Paediatric Teaching Hospital" *Australian Social Work* Vol 54, No 1 3-6

Nichols, CJ (1974) "The Silent Majority" *Australian Social Work* pp. 35-43

Nilsson, David (2004) Evaluating an International Leadership Program. Conference *paper delivered at the Doris Siegel Memorial Lecture, Mount Sinai Medical Center, New York, May 19, 2004*

O'Brien, L & Turner, C (1979) *Establishing Medical Social Work in Victoria,* University of Melbourne, Department of Social Studies, Victoria

Pockett, Rosalie (2003) "Staying in Hospital Social Work" *Social Work in Health Care* Vol 36 number 3 1-22

Rehr, H, Rosenberg, G, & Blumenfield S (1993) "Enhancing Leadership Skills through an International Exchange: The Mount Sinai Experience" *Social Work in Health Care,* Vol 18 3/4, 13-33

*Rendez-vous Quebec: Official Program: Fourth International Conference on Social Work in Health and Mental Health (2004)* University Laval, Quebec, Canada

Specht, H & Courtney, M E (1995) *Unfaithful Angels: How SocialWork has Abandoned its Mission* USA, Free Press

*The Origin and Development of Medical Social Work in Victoria, with Special Reference to the Work of the Victorian Institute of Hospital Almoners* (1951) Victoria, Australia

*The First International Conference on Social Work in Health and Mental Health Care* (1995) *Program and Abstract Book,* Hebrew University of Jerusalem Paul Baerwald School of Social Work, Jerusalem, Israel

*Visions from Around the Globe: 3rd International Conference on Social Work in Health and Mental Health: Abstracts (2001) Tampere, Finland*

Wee, A (2002) Social Work Education in Singapore: Early Beginnings in Tan Ngoh Tiong & Kalyani K. Mehta (eds) *Extending Frontiers Social Issues and Social Work in Singapore* Singapore, Eastern Universities Press

Weeks, W (1993*) Social Work and social Change: Professionalism in Social Work divergent class allegiances in the development of the profession* (unpublished teaching materials)

Weeks, W (undated) *Key Dates in Australian Social Work* (unpublished teaching materials)

Wolfensberger, W (1972) *Normalization: The principle of normalization in human services, National Institute on Mental Retardation,* Toronto

# The International Exchange Program:
# In the First Person

Nancy F. Cincotta, LCSW
Nicole Tokatlian, BA, BSW, DipMentHlthSc
Jane Miller, BA, DipSocStuds, MSW

**SUMMARY.** This commentary presents personal reflections on the Social Work Leadership Enhancement Program in the Department of Social Work Services at the Mount Sinai Medical Center in New York. The
value of the program, not only for the participants from other countries,
but also the value of the exposure of social workers from other countries
to the department staff is recognized. The international influence is un-
equalled. How if affects and nurtures global social work thinking, its impact on those taking part in the program, as well as the ever-expanding
influence of the program on a growing network of social workers is
noted. *[Article copies available for a fee from The Haworth Document Delivery
Service: 1-800-HAWORTH. E-mail address: <docdelivery@haworthpress.com>
Website: <http://www.HaworthPress.com> © 2006 by The Haworth Press, Inc. All
rights reserved.]*

---

Nancy F. Cincotta is Director of Psychosocial Services, Camp Sunshine, Casco,
Maine, and Bereavement Consultant, The Mount Sinai Hospital, New York. Nicole
Tokatlian is Senior Clinician/Team Leader, Haematology and Oncology Social Work
Team, and Co-Director of Psychosocial Services, Children's Cancer Centre Royal
Children's Hospital, Melbourne, Australia. Jane Miller is Director of Social Work,
Royal Children's Hospital, Melbourne, Australia.

[Haworth co-indexing entry note]: "The International Exchange Program: In the First Person." Cincotta,
Nancy F., Nicole Tokatlian, and Jane Miller. Co-published simultaneously in *Social Work in Health Care*
(The Haworth Press, Inc.) Vol. 43, No. 2/3, 2006, pp. 193-197; and: *International Social Health Care Policy,
Programs, and Studies* (ed: Gary Rosenberg, and Andrew Weissman) The Haworth Press, Inc., 2006, pp.
193-197. Single or multiple copies of this article are available for a fee from The Haworth Document Delivery
Service [1-800-HAWORTH, 9:00 a.m. - 5:00 p.m. (EST). E-mail address: docdelivery@haworthpress.com].

Available online at http://swhc.haworthpress.com
© 2006 by The Haworth Press, Inc. All rights reserved.
doi:10.1300/J010v43n02_13

**KEYWORDS.** Social work leadership, mentorship, global issues, exchange programs

Many 'tangible' things are presented in this publication to provoke thought, encourage academic pursuits, and to acknowledge components of the interchange among those involved in the Mount Sinai International Social Work Leadership Enhancement Program. There are many things we do as professionals and many areas in which we choose to gain expertise. Beyond our shared ethics, knowledge, and commitment, there are those things that influence and sustain us as social workers.

In the early days of the exchange program, as a manager in the Social Work Department at Mount Sinai, I came to know many of the participants. Often the discussions were of innovative programs or approaches at Mount Sinai or in the departments of the visitors. How could a certain program be replicated? What knowledge was transferable? All the discussions and activities were within the context of an ever-changing health care system.

In 1998 I had my first opportunity to consult in the Department of Social Work at the Royal Children's Hospital in Melbourne. That occasion, a more than hot day in Victoria, stays embedded in my mind. I had done a fair amount of teaching in this country, but this experience stood out. Here were social workers, beyond capable and committed, willing to come in on a Sunday to talk about clinical issues, not because they had to, but because there was an opportunity. It is within that element of opportunity, in which as an educator you compartmentalize your knowledge, knowing that your teaching time is limited, recognizing that if you want to make an impact, you must seize the moment.

Whether you are learning or teaching (which is actually always a combination of both), it is quite empowering, as a social worker in health care to realize that regardless of the country in which you work, social workers all speak the same language. You can problem-solve, reflect, and perhaps even understand your own accomplishments differently as you see them through the lens of those you set out to teach.

A dialogue that had begun in a conference room in New York came to life in a living room in Australia, continued at the Second International Conference on Social Work in Health and Mental Health in Melbourne and then on a professional road trip with Dr. Helen Rehr, from Melbourne to Adelaide and on to Sydney. Since that time, specialty social workers in oncology and bereavement programs have grown even more connected through many national social work organizations. As the exchange partnership evolved, so did email and the dialogue became easier to continue. The Doris Siegel Symposium was yet another place to affirm the connections, quickly followed by the Fourth International Conference on Social Work in Health and Mental Health in Quebec.

After sharing an office with four exchange social workers, I was honored to be invited to return to Australia this year. The lessons I learned on my journey were related to the cumulative experience of those willing to participate in the many professional engagements. The language used in working with children who are dying, the study of the use of hope in social work practice, who social workers are, what we do and how we approach our work, seemed to be tied together within this professional community. The energy derived from a cohort of social workers around the world working with people facing the same issues is boundless.

Part of what you learn from exposing yourself to an international community is that thinking globally affects what you do locally and working locally impacts what you teach and support globally.

The Mount Sinai Social Work Leadership Enhancement Program, founded by Dr. Helen Rehr, has led to a number of significant professional/collegial relationships. Social work in New York has had the advantage of having been established in heath care settings about thirty years earlier than in Australia and is delivered to a larger population base. American social work practitioners are graduates of more comprehensive education systems with post-graduate accreditation.

International participants in the Social Work Leadership Enhancement Program leave the program with a sense of "how things could work," a sense of potential, and of expansion. Through connections made within the program, several key social work leaders have been invited to Australia to provide educational forums and ongoing mentorship. Professor Irwin Epstein has visited Australia numerous times and is credited as being the catalyst for the launch of the practice-based research movement in health care social work. Dr. Susan Blumenfield, in her two visits to Australia and her commitment to the continuation of the Mount Sinai Social Work Leadership Enhancement Program, has provided ongoing mentorship for present and future social work directors and leaders. Virginia Walther's presentation to Victorian health care and welfare professionals was timely in profiling social work's role in working in intimate partner violence and she has subsequently acted as a consultant to senior police officials. Dr. Helen Rehr, serving as mentor, speaker, educator, coordinator, and more roles than can be identified, has been instrumental on both continents since the inception of the program.

International participants in the Mount Sinai program have been able to use their existing networks and connections in Australia, and their knowledge of the expertise of the Mount Sinai Department of Social Work, to facilitate study and education programs that have been of mutual benefit.

My second visit to Australia focused on clinical mentorship through a series of Grand Rounds and keynote addresses, presentations, and individual consultations. There was a local organizing committee, composed of key staff members of a number of hospitals, universities, and organizations that work with children with chronic and life-threatening illnesses and their families. Relationships formed through Mount Sinai, the International Social Work in Health and Mental Health conferences, meetings with workers from Australia at the Association of Pediatric Oncology Social Workers, as well as years of telephone and email correspondence, made this trip to Australia seem like part of a natural evolution.

Throughout the exchange program, cultural experiences and social events not only enhance relationships, but also allow discussion and thought about cultural differences and similarities. While the visits are obviously focused on professional endeavors, they are predicated on and consolidate a number of close professional friendships, which sustain and make possible the educational programs.

The cycle of exchange and relationship building continues. Several staff members from the various organizations will visit Camp Sunshine in Casco, Maine within twelve months of the visit to Australia. There are future plans in Australia for more in-depth, in-person consultation and teaching, as well as plans to continue consultation via telephone and teleconferencing. There are connections and reflections daily. Mine is but one of the several growing international partnerships.

Who we are as social work leaders and who we become are invariably influenced by the experiences we encounter along the way. It is comfortable to come to know your own skills as a practitioner, researcher, and manager within the context of your own environment. The exploration and refinement of those skills, and then sharing them in the professional arena is one way in which practice moves to theory and programs move to models.

It is within the context of the International Exchange Program while in Australia, that I come to understand that the excitement of shared work that can occur on two continents is about partnerships driven by common commitments to the universal issues facing the families with whom we have all chosen to work.

With each partnership and extension of the experience, the Mount Sinai International Leadership Program should receive accolades. It is one thing to bring together professionals to learn under your roof. It is another to watch them go out and grow and expand their knowledge beyond the walls of the institution. Many of the interactions in the exchange program allow social workers to value their roles as social workers, regardless of whether they are the travelers, the experts, or the professionals making connections on their home ground.

Although we are many years into it, the adventure of the journey of international interchange has only begun for many of us. For us, it has become a critical component of the way we think about social work practice. At the end of the day, the efforts of this program should be recognized as career-sustaining for many social work leaders who will have made an impact in many ways, large and small, and those which defy description.

# Psychiatry, Testimony, and Shoah:
# Reconstructing the Narratives of the Muted

Baruch Greenwald, MSW
Oshrit Ben-Ari, MSW
Rael D. Strous, MD
Dori Laub, MD

**SUMMARY.** A 1999 examination of approximately 5000 long-term psychiatric patients in Israel identified 725 as Holocaust (Shoah) survivors. Review of these cases has shown that these patients had not been treated as a unique group, and that their trauma-related illnesses had been neglected in their decades long treatment. We discovered that many of these patients had never openly shared their severe persecution history. We postulated that many of them could have avoided lengthy if not life-long psychiatric hospitalization had they been able to openly share that history. Instead, those gruesome and traumatic experiences remained encapsulated, split-off, causing the survivor to lead a double-life. These patients

---

Baruch Greenwald is Director of Social Services and Director of Holocaust Survivor Home, Beer Yaakov Mental Health Center, Beer Yaakov, Israel, and affiliated with the Sackler Faculty of Medicine, Tel-Aviv University. Oshrit Ben-Ari is Social Worker, Holocaust Survivor Home, Beer Yaakov, Israel. Rael D. Strous is Director of Chronic Inpatient Department, Beer Yaakov Mental Health Center, Beer Yaakov, Israel, and affiliated with the Sackler Faculty of Medicine, Tel-Aviv University. Dori Laub is Associate Professor, Department of Psychiatry, Yale University, New Haven, CT, USA.

Address correspondence to: Baruch Greenwald, MSW, Beer Yaakov Mental Health Center, P.O.B. 1, Beer Yaakov, 70350, Israel (E-mail: baruchng@yahoo.com).

[Haworth co-indexing entry note]: "Psychiatry, Testimony, and Shoah: Reconstructing the Narratives of the Muted." Greenwald, Baruch et al. Co-published simultaneously in *Social Work in Health Care* (The Haworth Press, Inc.) Vol. 43, No. 2/3, 2006, pp. 199-214; and: *International Social Health Care Policy, Programs, and Studies* (ed: Gary Rosenberg, and Andrew Weissman) The Haworth Press, Inc., 2006, pp. 199-214. Single or multiple copies of this article are available for a fee from The Haworth Document Delivery Service [1-800-HAWORTH, 9:00 a.m. - 5:00 p.m. (EST). E-mail address: docdelivery@haworthpress.com].

Available online at http://swhc.haworthpress.com
© 2006 by The Haworth Press, Inc. All rights reserved.
doi:10.1300/J010v43n02_14

may physically inhabit the world as psychogeriatric patients, though emotionally they may remain in adolescence or childhood due to early traumatic experiences. Some twenty-six patients at two institutions gave consent to be interviewed by a professional team and have their testimonies recorded on videotape. The aim of this study was to investigate the role of video testimony as a potential useful psychotherapeutic clinical intervention. By videotaping testimonies of these patients' experiences before, during, and after World War II, we had created highly condensed texts that could be interpreted on a multiplicity of levels going far beyond the mere narrative content of clinical medical history. Joint observation, reiteration, and discussion of these testimonies with staff members and the patients themselves has been not only an interesting experience, but also one of therapeutic value yet to be fully appreciated. *[Article copies available for a fee from The Haworth Document Delivery Service: 1-800-HAWORTH. E-mail address: <docdelivery@haworthpress.com> Website: <http://www.Haworth Press. com> © 2006 by The Haworth Press, Inc. All rights reserved.]*

KEYWORDS. Psychiatric, Israel, Holocaust (Shoah) survivors, testimonies

## INTRODUCTION

Out of a group of about 5,000 long-term psychiatric patients hospitalized in Israel since 1999, a disproportionate number of about 725 were identified as Holocaust survivors (Bazak Commission, 1999). A review of these cases showed that these patients had not been treated as a unique group, and that their trauma-related illnesses had been neglected in their decades-long treatment. Most of these patients had been diagnosed as having chronic schizophrenia, with no special attention given to the historical circumstances related to their psychiatric symptoms and disabilities. Many of the psychiatrists that treated them insist today that these patients do not respond to traditional treatment such as anti-psychotic medication (Cahn, 1995; Riess, 2002). We postulated that many of them could have avoided lengthy if not life-long psychiatric hospitalization, had they been able or had an opportunity in their careers, or by society at large to more openly share their severe history of persecution. Instead, those gruesome and traumatic experiences remain encapsulated and split-off, causing the survivor to lead a double life. These patients may physically inhabit the world as geriatrics, though emotionally, they may remain fixed in adolescence. Thus, the aim of this study was to investigate the role of video testimony as a potential useful clinical intervention many years after the acute traumatic event and to analyze the content of the video testimony for clinical material which may be useful in the psychotherapeutic process with the patient.

## METHOD

### Study Population

The study population consisted of chronic in-patients at two large state referral institutions in Israel. The subjects were drawn from the approximately 100 residents (age range of 59-97 years) housed in the hostel section for Holocaust survivors established in 2000, all of whom have severe, chronic mental illness. For study inclusion, subjects met criteria as victims of Nazi persecution as defined by the Conference on Jewish Claims Against Germany, Inc. (in hiding, ghettos, concentration labor and death camps, etc.), who were at least 3 years old during the time of persecution, and who were willing and capable of telling a story. Survivors were excluded if they exhibited features of major cognitive impairment or severe psychotic disorganization that would preclude video testimony participation. The study was approved by the local Helsinki Committee Ethical Review Committee and the Yale Human Investigation Committee. Subjects and their legal guardians provided signed informed consent once the nature of the study and its potential risks and benefits were fully explained. Consent was also obtained from the subject's designated clinician. In addition to the right to terminate participation at any time during the study, subjects were informed they had the right to prohibit the sharing of video testimony and to withdraw it at any time from the Video Archive or the locked collections for future medical training and research.

### Video Testimony

For the purposes of documenting and studying these experiences, 26 patients were recruited and interviewed by mental health professionals. Their testimonies were recorded on videotape. In addition to the video testimony, they also participated in a psychiatric evaluation and psychological testing. By videotaping testimonies of these patients' experiences before, during, and after World War II, we created highly condensed texts that could be interpreted on multiple levels going far beyond the mere narrative content of clinical medical history. We believed that severe psychological trauma could be better addressed through the medium of video testimony. Joint observation, reiteration, and discussion of these testimonies with staff members and the patients, themselves, have proven to be an interesting and important experience. This has been accomplished by means of an individual one by one careful and precise analysis of form and content of the clinical interview. We have addressed the issue of whether or not massive psychic trauma is related to severe chronic mental illness with a psychotic disability that leads to chronic or multiple psychiatric hospitalizations. For example, patients that had been diagnosed for years as suffering from schizophrenia might have been more correctly diagnosed as having Post Traumatic Stress Disorder, which was related to their World War II experiences, and had this been the case, the entire course of treatment might have been altered. Although we know that this diagnostic entity (PTSD) was not in existence as such in the 1950s and 1960s, know-how about PTSD symptoms was already commencing at this time and the diagnostic entity itself has been in the DSM for over 20 years. Likewise, we questioned whether a therapeutic intervention such as a video testimony, which helps build a narrative for the traumatic experience and gives it coherent expression, might help in alleviating the symptoms of the disorder and thus change its course. Whether these changes may be attributed to direct intervention through the patient's testimony or are a result of an indirect intervention through planning treatment, involvement with family members or the survivor community, or the knowledge that the videotaped testimony will be made available to others, is an open question.

During the course of each of the 26 testimony interviews, emphasis was placed on a cooperative reconstruction of a continuous life history containing pre-Holocaust experiences entrapped sometimes in a vague, ambiguous past, a description of the patients' own subjective Holocaust experience, post-World War II experiences until the present, and an attempt to understand what significant role the patients' tragic past plays in their life today. Through this reconstruction, the mourning process is able to take place and hopefully be alleviated. In the years of turmoil and upheaval following World War II, there was often no opportunity to be involved in such a mourning process. The patients were involved in immigrating to a new country (often illegally), fighting for survival, trying to rebuild families, and learning vocations. If one desired to share with others details of their misfortunate past and degrading experiences, neither the layperson nor professional would legitimatize then what we would view today as a therapeutic as well as a humane necessity. Their experiences were too horrendous for members of today's society to absorb. During the testimony interview, steps had to be taken to aid the subjects in restoring that very sense of self that had been dealt such a devastating blow in both the Holocaust and the upheaval thereafter. In the testimony interviews, we attempt to create a narrative that is both detailed and organized, by utilizing cognitive, affective, and sensory elements. The cognitive channel emphasizes a detailed reconstruction of historical facts related to the traumatic events, the affective channel reconstructs feelings then and now, and the sensory channel reconstructs bodily sensations, sights, smells, and sounds. The testimonial experience is a collaborative venture, since the interviewer assumes the position of a companion or compassionate chronicler of a journey into the self and into the past, a journey without any complete pre-existing conscious map of the territory to be uncovered. The document created is intended to be a permanent one for posterity, preserved as a virtual or real record in a safe place. It also serves to affirm facts that the victims either were unable to relate to, or the facts were known but the victims were prevented from telling, or simply did not dare express before the testimonial event.

The video testimony process began with a preliminary impression of the subject's persecution history, gained from either his personal file or a pre-interview, after acquiring permission from the patient and guardian, and responding to any questions and concerns about the subject. A team of two interviewers and a video technician took each testimony. These three individuals were usually outsiders, not previously acquainted with the subjects. Past experience with testimonies have indicated that the victims' pre-existing transference feelings toward people in the interview may impede them in testifying freely and in an unencumbered fashion. The average video session lasted about 60 to 90 minutes. The processed films, which were not edited and contained the contents of the entire sessions, became available to us about six weeks after the initial interviews. After the staff director had viewed the films, individual staff members were invited to sit with the patient and view the testimony together (with the patient's permission). In two cases, the patients objected at first, but agreed later after other patients had finished joint video sessions. The viewing event lasted for one or two sessions, depending on the length of the particular testimony. After the joint viewing, staff members discussed the content with the patient. As a result of these meetings, the staff felt enriched by learning about and vicariously experiencing the patient's life experiences. Consequently, a new and deeper bond was created between the staff and the patients, based on a mutual understanding of the tragic events that played such a major role in the patient's life and pathology. During the joint viewings, we were surprised that a number of the patients could not recognize themselves as the image giving the testimony on the screen. For example, patients said: 'Who is that?' or 'How does she know about that? Who told her?' What possible explanations might there be for this phenomenon? Perhaps viewing the images of themselves as encapsulated adolescents conflicted with their present views of themselves and they were unable to understand what had happened to themselves in the intervening years.

## TESTIMONIES

While all of the 26 clinical interviews yielded important and fascinating clinical material, the examples of Sarah, David, and Chana (aliases) have been chosen in particular here to illustrate the principal and impact of the testimonial experience. David's silent nature, as well as Sarah's and Chana's general anxiety and fear of leaving the premises of the Holocaust survivor unit could now be viewed in light of severely traumatic events that took place in their early adolescence.

Sarah was born in Greece in 1927, the second of three daughters. A year later, the family was uprooted to Belgium, where her father took a position as Rabbi of a Sephardic community. She had to leave school at the age of twelve and was hidden by others for almost two years in her own home in Nazi-controlled Belgium with her mother and two sisters, who bribed and bartered for survival, only to be eventually turned over to the Nazis by members of the local population and shipped to Auschwitz, where they were separated from their mother, whom they never saw again. The three surviving sisters returned to Belgium after the war, and while attempting to immigrate to Palestine in 1947, they were arrested by the British and held in a camp in Cyprus until they were allowed to immigrate a year later. Arriving in the newborn State of Israel, all three sisters settled on a kibbutz. Sarah describes the death of her older sister from pneumonia, as a result of the severe winter of 1950 (that winter, snow accumulated in most of Israel, the only time in the 20th century). Both of the two remaining sisters married and left the kibbutz for city life. We know of Sarah's subsequent divorce, described by her as a result of her unwillingness to become pregnant and bear children, due to her anxiety. She first began to receive care in a psychiatric outpatient clinic at the age of 34. After her divorce, she lived with her younger sister and her husband and helped care for their three children, until her first hospitalization at age 41 (1968). The reason for her hospitalization was anxiety; the diagnosis was "schizophrenic reaction." Sarah was in and out of several psychiatric hospitals for about three years, after which she was permanently hospitalized. In 1974, at the age of 47, she was sent by the Ministry of Health to a privately run institution. The Ministry opted to close this particular institute toward the end of 1999, after a parliamentary commission investigating the plight of the mentally afflicted Holocaust survivors in Israel found the conditions in this and several other institutions to be appalling (Bazak, 1999). Sarah was then moved to a new Holocaust Survivor Home, not a hospital itself, though located next to the campus of a psychiatric center. The filming of the testimonies took place at the survivor unit. Here are excerpts from Sarah's testimony:

### Excerpt 1

Interviewer: Where did they (the Nazis) find you?

Sarah: At home.

I: In your home?

S: Yes, in our home where we hid.

I: Where did you hide in your home?

S: In our own home. They forgot us. They forgot us for two years. Then someone informed them that there were still some Jews in some of the homes. They came to our house, and the first time they let us alone was under the condition that we would never tell anyone they had been there. Two weeks later other Nazis came and took us.

I: Who were the members of your family who hid there?

S: Me, my mother, and my two sisters. I told you, my father had already died of a heart attack. He took all our troubles "to heart" literally. He died on a Friday.

I: Was that after the war began?

S: Yes. You see my father was a Zaddik (righteous man). He got the (heart) attack on Friday (Sabbath eve) and the funeral was on Saturday.

I: Sarah, how were you able to get food while you were hiding in your house?

S: There was a black market. (This) man had a grocery store. It wasn't kosher, but he brought us food we could eat, good stuff. We paid him a lot of money. Thank God my mother had two heavy gold bracelets. She sold them for a lot of money. We were lucky, we bought eggs, yellow cheese, white cheese, jam, and white bread.

I: You paid him and he brought it to your home?

S: Yes, he brought (food) every night.

I: He wasn't a Jew?

S: Of course not, he was a Christian. He brought us food and got paid well for his services. He did it for the money. We were lucky. We had money because my mother sold her jewelry.

I: Where was your hiding place? What did it look like?

S: It was our own home. They forgot us. So we lived.

I: You mean they forgot you because there had already been searches and most of the Jews had been deported?

S: Yes, of course. They forgot us!

I: How was it that they forgot you, wasn't your home near (the other Jewish homes)?

S: No! They had a list of homes, our home was not on the list. They forgot us! That was our luck. If not, we would have been taken with all the others.

I: How did you live your lives in hiding for those two years? What was it like together? How was life during the day, during the night?

S: We lived in constant fear.

I: You were always scared?

S: Yes, we were always scared that they would come and take us. In the end, they were informed and they really did come and get us.

I: Did you ever leave the house (during the two years)?

S: No, never. Can you imagine it? For two years we never left the house. There was always fear that at any second they would come and take us. (sighs) I've been through so much in my life. I was also (imprisoned) in Cyprus.

## Excerpt 2

I: How did they find you at home?

S: They were informed. Some children told them in Flemish "There are still some Jews in that house." Can you imagine how we felt? They betrayed us. But still, the first time they came to our house they let us stay, on the condition that we would never tell anyone we had been there. Some of the Belgians were good.

I: Those who came, were they Nazis or Belgians?

S: One was a Nazi, one was a Belgian policeman.

I: Those who came and took you in the end, were they Nazis or Belgians?

S: Nazis, of course.

I: What did they look like?

S: Like Nazis, *Oy Veh* (oh my goodness!). They looked like demons!

I: Were they in uniform?

S: Yes, with swastikas. I saw the same ones at Auschwitz. They came with dogs.

I: Where did they take you?

S: They took us to a police station near Antwerp. There we joined the other groups who were transported to Auschwitz.

I: In trucks?

S: First we were in a jail. Before the trip to Auschwitz (when they came to our house) they took my mother and sister first. We remained in the house. They told us they would return soon to take us. I asked them if they would let us have coffee. They said, "Coffee will be waiting for you downstairs." I believed them. "Coffee" was the trip to Auschwitz.

I: The Nazi said. "Coffee will be waiting for you." This is important. They cheated you.

S: Yes, and now I will be getting reprimands from Germany. My sister already received them.

I: A truck was there for you downstairs?

S: Yes, they took us (to the station). There we were put on a train. They took us all, standing, in a cattle car. Three days. Three nights. Poor mother. Can you imagine? It was an open cattle car. Three days and three nights till we arrived (at Auschwitz). There they separated us from Mother. We never saw her again.

Many of the staff had not been aware of Sarah's hiding during the war, and even those of us who knew her history were not always aware of the intensity of her experiences during the entire war and thereafter. All we know about Sarah's psychiatric history supports a consistent picture of anxiety related to traumatic experience. Psychiatric testing before her testimony indicated PTSD symptoms. Sarah rarely ventures outside the premises of the Home, and on rare occasions when the staff had succeeded in convincing her to participate in outings, she was tense all the time, even screaming, for example, when the bus hit a bump, or if there were sudden noises. The night staff reported that Sarah still has nightmares about her experiences at Auschwitz. On the premises of the Home, Sarah is an active participant in all activities; she has a tendency to criticize staff members who may not meet all her immediate requests and has developed a dependent, sometimes symbiotic relationship with her roommate. The roommate, a younger woman who was a small child at the end of the Holocaust, grew up as an orphan, and some of her current psychotic content is the delusion that Sarah is really her mother. However, Sarah is not delusional or psychotic today. We think that her 1968 diagnosis of having a "schizophrenic reaction" is dubious and wonder how her life might have changed had she been given more appropriate treatment in the community, with behavioral therapy for anxiety, instead of being hospitalized all her life.

David, born in Czechoslovakia in 1934, was the younger of two siblings. We know that David began elementary school around 1940, already a time of turmoil. It was reported that he was an excellent pupil, very pedantic in his studies. The "normal" life of the family was soon interrupted by the war and the Holocaust, since they were able to survive only by hiding in bunkers for four, perhaps five years. Four years after the war (1949), the family immigrated to Israel, where David completed his high-school matriculation as well as army duty. In the army he had disciplinary problems and was discharged before serving his full term of duty. His first psychiatric hospitalization was in 1957, two years after his discharge from the army. His complaints then included anxiety and somatic symptoms. Like Sarah, he was hospitalized "on and off" in government-run hospitals for several years until he was permanently hospitalized in 1965 at the age of 31 in the same privately run institution that was closed in 1999, when David also moved to the new Holocaust Survivor's Home.

David was a very quiet man who never said more than two or three words. All that we knew about him was from his file or his elderly aunt. At first he refused to participate in the interview. However, soon after he suddenly said: "okay, lets do it!" He said little and most of the interview consisted of the interviewer speaking, to which he agreed or disagreed. David had no real memories of those years spent in the bunkers, only of asking his mother: "Why are we here?" He can't remember what she answered. When asked whether he felt terror all the time, his answer was "Probably." His facial and body expressions did speak of terror and sadness, yet he refused to acknowledge that he felt something. David was one of the only patients in the survivor's unit almost constantly silent but prone to violent outbursts if and when he felt his private space had been violated. This silent nature, which perhaps characterizes as many as 20% of the hospitalized psychiatric survivors, has its own uniqueness. These patients seem to walk around, intently observe, smoke, and then unexpectedly walk away. Some seem to be in a conflict or in a struggle when trying to pronounce a word. Even in interviews with many of the survivors that did talk, many deny memories of the Holocaust or simply use code words like "It was awful, you know" or "What is there to talk about?" David also viewed his testimony video together with staff members but had no verbal reactions to the film. Apparently, David had been suffering, and he died unexpectedly four months after his testimony, of massive, undiagnosed lung cancer.

Chana's videotaped testimony was shown at the Fourth International Conference on Social work in Health and Mental Health in Quebec in May, 2004. Chana had agreed to our showing of her film to an overseas audience, yet we have abided by her request not to show it to her son. Interestingly, a day after giving her permission, she appeared in the director's office urgently requesting that a copy of the film remain in Israel should her son wish to view it in the future. We calmed her, explaining that that we have two copies of the film: one intended for the researchers and a second one, her copy, which has also remained in our hands at her request. Usually the second copy is given to a guardian or family member after permission from the patient.

Chana was born in a village in eastern Romania in 1927, the youngest child in a family of five siblings. Shortly after the war began, the family was forcibly uprooted and moved to the primarily Jewish town of Yasi. Chana remained in Yasi after the war, wed, bore a child, and divorced, all before immigrating to Israel in 1948. In Israel she lived with her sister and son, wed again, and divorced again after a second son. She was already showing signs of so-called mental illness, and did not raise her second son, with whom she has been separated ever since. From information we have in her file, self-neglect and behavior described as unusual or bizarre preceded psychiatric hospitalizations. Diagnosed as having paranoid schizophrenia, she was in and out of hospitals until the Health Ministry authorized her permanent hospitalization in the same previously mentioned privately run institution in 1980. She also moved to the Holocaust Survivor's Home when the private institution was closed.

### Excerpt 1

Interviewer: Can you remember the massacre of Jews that took place in Yasi?

Chana: It was. It was. My father buried maybe a thousand victims. He dug a huge pit.

I: Your father?

C: (My) father. Dug a huge pit and dropped the bodies. They were naked. They came from the Death Train. Daddy had to take the corpses. I think, I remember I helped him; we put them on a wagon. We carried them to the pit.

I: In Yasi 30,000 Jews were killed at the beginning (of the war).

C: It was. I forgot how you call it. A massacre.

I: A massacre of the Jews. A huge pogrom. And they called your father to come and help bury (the dead).

C: Yes.

I: They took children (to help bury)?

C: Yes, they took. The Germans came and forced us. They said, "schneller! *schneller!*"(Faster, faster).

I: Can you remember how the Germans looked?

C: I remember how they looked.

I: How did they look?

C: They had green forest uniforms.

I: As a child . . .

C: 12 years old

I: Yes, 12 years old, you yourself already had to bury corpses. How did that affect you?

C: It instilled in me fear. A deep fear. A fear of death. (sighs)

## *Excerpt 2*

C: Suddenly there was an alarm. Airplanes came to bomb us. We did not know whether or not to run to the bunker. I stayed in the house. They all ran to the bunker. We had an old grandmother, mother's mother. My sister took her. I stayed alone in the house. Then the bombing began. I did not know whether or not I should run to the bunker. I was afraid if I stayed in the house it would collapse on me. I did not know what to do. Then I decided to run to the bunker. Shrapnel fell near my leg. I did not know whether to continue running or stay where I was in the middle of the street.

I: So you ran to the bunker?

C: Yes, I ran to the bunker. I did not know what to do, to run or stay where I was. Afterwards a bomb fell (directly) on the second bunker next to us. Everyone was buried; we dug ourselves out with our hands.

I: Everyone was buried?

C: Yes.

I: You were in the bunker when this happened?

C: Yes, I was there.

I: During the bombing?

C: We all sought refuge.

I: The bunker collapsed, but you all got out.

C: (agrees)

## *Excerpt 3*

C: (sighs) It's hard to remember all of this.

I: It's hard to remember. Do these pictures come back even when you don't want (to think about it)?

C: I have dreams about it. But then I realize that, thank God, we are here now, free. It's a great miracle. But they shouldn't throw us out of here as well. I think about it. Maybe they will close down this place and throw us out, who knows where! (pause, then looking straight at the interviewer) Will they close this place?

I: No, never.

After viewing Chana's testimony in its entirety, the staff members can now more easily recognize the connection between Chana's traumatic childhood, her suspicious behavior, lack of trust, self-neglect, and inability to make independent decisions or even be critical. However, this does not seem to be due to a lack of affect as a negative symptom of schizophrenia. She currently has no delusional behavior. Her psychiatric testing before the testimony indicates both PTSD and some symptoms of psychosis, with a slight decrease in the post-test. What we observe on a daily basis is a sad, older lady, who, in the course of her lifetime has experienced uprooting from place to place, mostly unwilling, village-to-village, country-to-country, until she reached the Survivor Home. Even at the Survivor Home, she tends to define for herself what she considers as a "safe" territory, often standing at the entrance to her room and leaving only to go to the dining room at meal times or when a staff member calls her for a specific activity. Before the taping of the testimonies, it was known that Chana never attended outings organized by the staff, including concerts, movies, or one-day trips. During 2004, a student, under our close supervision, worked intensely with Chana, making every effort to gain her trust and to get her to join her in attending both inside and outside activities, with only partial success. Unfortunately, the tense security and terror situation in Israel has added to Chana's insecurity. The staff members found her last remarks in the testimony both genuine and sad: "Will they throw us out of here and throw us who knows where?"

## CONCLUSIONS

Since we are dealing with patients who have been institutionalized for 20-30 years and more, we need to properly characterize them today not only as Holocaust survivors, but also as survivors of psychiatric hospitalization. As a result, many of these patients have undergone a process of institutionalization and lost interest in life outside the hospital surroundings. Impressions that we have collected, from both those patients videotaped and those not, support changing the sole diagnosis of schizophrenia, which was assigned for years to many of the mentally afflicted survivors. We may be dealing with a long-term PTSD with psychotic features, in some cases. We are well aware of the fact that survivors previously unable to discuss their traumatic past are now forming new bonds with staff members, who, as a result of the survivors' testimonies, are much more aware of the patients' history. A therapeutic group, using both the contents of the testimonies and other reminiscing techniques, has provided new venues for self-expression, and even the social outings of the patients have now taken on a new significance, since staff members have been able to convince some of the previously immobile residents to participate. Knowing and understanding their past has made its impact. Realizing that as a result of the Holocaust trauma, the individual's very sense of self was very often erased, we are attempting to take steps to restore that self, by enabling more self-expression and encouraging empowerment.

## REFERENCES

Bazak,Y. (1999), The Findings of the Public Committee of Inquiry into the Situation of the Psychiatrically Ill Patients Hospitalized in Israeli Psychiatric Facilities (Hebrew, available from the Israeli Ministry of Health). The committee was composed of parliamentary members, government ministers, and experts in the field.

Cahn, D. (1995), Holocaust Survivors Mistreated, Associated Press release, November 26, 1995.

Rees, M. (2002), Surviving the Past, Time Magazine, January 14, 2002.

# Index

© 2006 by The Haworth Press, Inc. All rights reserved.

T - #0524 - 101024 - C0 - 212/152/13 - PB - 9780789033482 - Gloss Lamination